Breast Cancer and the Post-Surgical Body

Breast Cancer and the Post-Surgical Body

Recovering the Self

Samantha Crompvoets

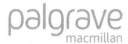

First published 2006 by
PALGRAVE MACMILLAN
Houndmills, Basingstoke, Hampshire RG21 6XS and
175 Fifth Avenue, New York, N.Y. 10010
Companies and representatives throughout the world

PALGRAVE MACMILLAN is the global academic imprint of the Palgrave
Macmillan division of St. Martin's Press, LLC and of Palgrave Macmillan Ltd.
Macmillan® is a registered trademark in the United States, United Kingdom
and other countries. Palgrave is a registered trademark in the European
Union and other countries.

ISBN-13: 978–1–4039–9900–9 hardback
ISBN-10: 1–4039–9900–7 hardback

This book is printed on paper suitable for recycling and made from fully
managed and sustained forest sources.

A catalogue record for this book is available from the British Library.

Library of Congress Cataloging-in-Publication Data
Crompvoets, Samantha, 1976–
    Breast cancer and the post-surgical body : recovering the self / Samantha
    Crompvoets.
      p.   cm.
    Includes bibliographical references and index.
    ISBN 1–4039–9900–7 (cloth)
    1. Breast—Cancer—Psychological aspects.   I. Title.
    [DNLM: 1. Breast Neoplasms—psychology.   2. Mastectomy—
    psychology.   3. Body Image.   4. Feminism.   5. Mammaplasty—
    psychology.   6. Self Concept.   WP 870 C945b 2006]
    RC280.B8C76 2006
    616.99′4490019—dc22   2005058645

10   9   8   7   6   5   4   3   2   1
15   14   13   12   11   10   09   08   07   06

Printed and bound in Great Britain by
Antony Rowe Ltd, Chippenham and Eastbourne

For Timothy, Joseph and Zara

Contents

List of Tables and Figures

Tables

Figures

Acknowledgements

Foremost, I wish to thank the many women who participated in this study. I am indebted to them for the time, honesty and friendship they gave me. In particular, I would like to thank Jenny Mendick and Felicity Lehmann for their enthusiasm and insight. I warmly acknowledge the support and encouragement of Dorothy Broom, Andrea Whittaker, Anni Dugdale and Kevin White. Finally, thanks to Tim, Joseph and Zara for never letting me lose sight of the bigger picture.

Acronyms and Abbreviations

ABA	Australian Broadcasting Authority
ACT	Australian Capital Territory (also known as Canberra)
AMA	American Medical Association
ASB	Advertising Standards Bureau
ASPS	American Society of Plastic Surgeons
AWHN	Australian Women's Health Network
BCAG	Breast Cancer Action Group
BCNA	Breast Cancer Network Australia
BCSS	Breast Cancer Support Service
Bilat	Bilateral Mastectomy
Chemo	Chemotherapy
CTFA	Cosmetic, Toiletry and Fragrance Association
CV	Curriculum Vitae
GP	General Practitioner
HRT	Hormone Replacement Therapy
LGFB	Look Good . . . Feel Better
MRS	Mastectomy Rehabilitation Services
NBCC	National Breast Cancer Centre
NBCF	National Breast Cancer Foundation
NH&MRC	National Health and Medical Research Council
NSW	New South Wales
TRAM Flap	Transverse Rectus Abdominal Muscle Flap reconstruction
UK	United Kingdom
USA	United States of America
VIC	Victoria

1
An Unacceptable Body

Introduction

In October 1998 Breast Cancer Awareness Month was brought to the Australian public's attention through a controversial advertising campaign. The focus of the campaign was a commercial featuring a prominent public relations consultant and ex-actress, Barbara Joss, revealing her mastectomy scar. Not wanting to be identified at the time, the images of Ms Joss are from the neck down, her torso covered initially in a pink, lacy bed jacket with a bow at the neck (Figure 1.1). The advertisement begins with a side profile of Ms Joss's torso, her hand at her neck. The male voice-over reads: 'They say showing a woman's pair of breasts...will help get people's attention.' She then turns to face the camera, her hand unties the bow and she pushes the jacket aside to reveal her right breast. The voice-over continues: 'we thought showing just one would work better'. Ms Joss then pushes away the other side of her jacket revealing the site of her mastectomy.

Three versions of the advertisement were shot, with the campaign writers concerned that the commercials were probably too explicit to get passed by the Australian Broadcasting Authority (ABA) and Advertising Standards Bureau (ASB). Ms Joss had to audition for the advertisement, which involved having the director and his personal assistant visit her at home shortly after the mastectomy and view her post-surgical body. They had many women willing to do the advertisement but they wanted someone with a 'slight' body, a larger woman's one-breasted torso considered 'unappetizing'.[1]

Although fear campaigns always elicit mixed responses and are labeled 'controversial' there are no records of complaints from the public being made to either the ABA or the ASB. There are also no records of

1

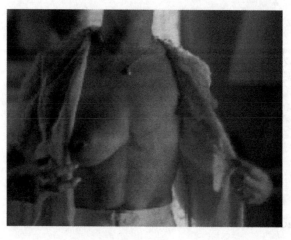

Figure 1.1 National Breast Cancer Foundation advertisement for Breast Cancer Awareness Month, October 1998. Still courtesy of Jack Watts Currie Advertising Agency.

complaints being made to the advertising agency who scripted the campaign (Jack Watts Currie) or the National Breast Cancer Foundation (NBCF) which funded it.

Surprisingly, negative responses to the campaign came only from breast cancer organizations, with BreastScreen NSW (New South Wales) leading the push to have the advertisement taken off air. Concerned that the advertisements would frighten women from being screened, BreastScreen argued that it was a fear campaign portraying the outcome of only a minority of women with breast cancer. They also had concerns for the minority it did depict – how would these women feel about others knowing how their mastectomized bodies really looked? Professor Sally Redman, Director of the National Breast Cancer Centre (NBCC), went on *A Current Affair*, a prime time current affairs programme, denigrating the use of 'shock tactics' and arguing that such a 'graphic depiction' would only discourage women from attending mammographic screening.[2] Prior to the campaign's release a large faction of the NBCF attempted to stop it going ahead, arguing along similar lines.

Featuring in the campaign days after starting chemotherapy, Barbara Joss describes the experience as nerve-racking and the difficulties she had 'baring a terrible body'.[3] She says she was frightened to look at the mastectomy site but felt indebted to the screening process which saved her life. Her motivation then was to help spread the word, that breast cancer kills 1 in 11 women and that funds are needed for research. Her body was testimony to the devastation caused by a terrible disease.

Soon after the campaign aired Ms Joss 'came out', identifying herself to be the mastectomized torso in the controversial advertisement. Her illness experience was detailed in a feature story in *Woman's Day* Magazine[4] and she appeared on *The Midday Show with Kerri-Anne Kennerley*.[5] The interviews were used as a springboard to discuss the importance of breast cancer awareness and research and applauded Barbara's bravery at revealing her post-surgical body.

The M-rated advertisement was controversial in two ways: first because it showed a mastectomy scar, and secondly, because it went against the popular soft image of breast cancer campaigns. The Jack Watts Currie Advertising Agency were keen to run the advertisement again in 1999, but the NBCF decided that this was not the image of their organization they wanted to project. Instead the public face of breast cancer was to be a myriad of celebrity 'ambassadors' who are largely personally unaffected by breast cancer.

Ms Joss went on to have her breast surgically reconstructed, and her autobiographical narrative was later published in her book *My Left Breast* (1999). Ms Joss's transformation from the mastectomized body in the advertisement to one which she considered 'whole again' was detailed heavily, producing a recovery trajectory that balanced the initial confronting images of her amputated breast and offered a sense of hope that all could be restored. In her book she likens her un-reconstructed body to a Christmas present, having pretty wrapping and tinsel and bows, a façade that could be taken away revealing the 'truth' about her incomplete body. For Barbara, the only way she was able to accept what had happened was to have a reconstruction.

The campaign raises many questions: Why is the sight of a mastectomized body so unacceptable? In the face of such high-profile opposition, how can the mastectomized body ever become normalized? Can women ever reclaim a 'complete' self in the absence of a breast or breasts?

The Barbara Joss advertisement symbolizes the tensions that exist between the post-surgical body and self. As women attempt to come to grips with the changed landscape of their mastectomized body and the challenges a breast cancer crisis has brought to their sense of self, they are simultaneously faced with powerful social discourses which situate their body as incomplete, abnormal and unfeminine without two breasts. Furthermore, the restoration of their health and well-being is positioned as intricately linked to regaining their pre-surgery appearance. The absence of a public and a private discourse which frames the mastectomized body positively demands critical attention as it impedes an embodied recovery from breast cancer.

This book is concerned with the lived experience of the mastectomized body, bringing a sensitivity to the micropolitics of breast cancer organizations and the political economy of breast restoration. It is contextualized in a broad sociological framework, and speaks to theories of phenomenology of illness experience, narrative construction of identity, feminism and the body, and the politics of health.

This research examines the post-surgical body and the construction and reconstruction of this body in the context of breast cancer. I am interested in how the body is negotiated, constituted, mobilized and performed by and for women with breast cancer. I explore how the mastectomized body and self is constituted in language, in the stories that women tell about their illness experience, and in practice, how both words and things perform the post-surgical body in particular ways.

I argue that the current treatment of the post-surgical body within breast cancer culture and wider society allows no space for women to reconceptualize their bodies as normal, feminine or complete in the absence of a breast or breasts. Instead, the mastectomized body is positioned as transient, to be 'fixed' as soon as possible. I argue that breast restoration, wearing a prosthesis or surgical reconstruction, is presented as the only mechanism available for women to renegotiate a complete sense of self.

My initial interest in breast cancer and the post-surgical body elicited many questions that this study addresses: What are the patterns in women's accounts of breast surgery? Are there any? What are the different discourses of breast surgery? What questions do they ask? What do they reveal? How do different discourses and narratives define and mobilize normality, identity and sexuality? What are the tropes that enable the stability of these definitions and narratives? How is this knowledge legitimated? How do the microparticulars of women's accounts fit with macrocultural structures? How does breast reconstruction fit with feminist ideology?

At one level this research moves beyond individual experiences to examine the politics of choices that women are given and what constrains and influences those choices. I do not want to deny the experiences of women who are happy with their restored breasts, nor I am trying to undermine the positive experiences women have had. As a woman who has not had breast cancer, I am unable to share the experience. Rather I am indebted to the thoughts, feelings, emotions and insights of the women I interviewed which enabled the making of this book.

The study of the post-surgical body is crucial to furthering our understanding of the corporeality of breast cancer and enabling more sensitive and practical approaches to rehabilitating women during and after their illness experience.

Entering the field

I came away from my first interview stunned at how deeply affected I was by what had just been shared with me, overwhelmed by the openness and depth of information and emotion, quite unsure as to what I should have done when the participant broke down in tears, and how I should have responded when she hugged me as I left her house. Before I 'entered the field' my expectations of the interview process were that I would have an open discussion with the participant about her experience, with her taking me through her account in an order that was significant to her. I expected there to be a lot of emotion from both myself and the participant, and for some women that this may be the first time they had articulated their experience. I am not sure how, or if in fact at all, I could have better prepared myself for this process.

The ethics application required as part of my doctoral work was an opportunity to clarify the aims and objectives of my study and think through any problems that could arise in the data collection. Cannon (1989) highlights the significance of involvement, detachment and personal responsibility when studying topics of an emotive nature. She argues that the importance of the emotional presence of the researcher in the interview setting is critical to the development of an open and shared relationship with the respondent. Similarly, Oakley (1981) believes that the interviewer should invest her own personal identity in the research relationship by answering respondents questions, sharing knowledge and experience and giving support when asked. For me this was not something of which I had to be consciously aware; instead it was implicit in the research process. Both the focus of the research and the methods of inquiry demanded a level of personal involvement from myself as a researcher. In no way did I intend to come to the interview as the all-knowing researcher ready to 'make sense' of someone's story. Instead it was a shared experience, the participant making sense and ordering her experience through her narrative and me as a researcher able to draw from it what I thought the participant emphasized as major themes. In line with Cotterill (1992) I argue that the interview is a fluid encounter where balances of power, control and vulnerability are not fixed between researcher and respondent. Instead balances shift between and during different interview situations.

One of the primary aims of this research is to make women's experiences visible and render them legitimate forms of knowledge. Thus I want to explore subjugated knowledges, that is experiential knowledge.

In my ethics application I described how if a woman became distressed during the interview I would give her the details of local support groups and counsellors and the number for Life Line. Not being a trained counsellor myself I saw this as the most appropriate and professional response. However, after sharing such intimate details of her life and illness many questions concerned me: What was my responsibility to this woman now as she had told me more than she had told even her partner? How was I to acknowledge this bond if I saw her again? As I left the house, was I a researcher or a friend? I felt the translation from one to the other had been made in the course of the interview, and in fact had enabled the interview. What was my commitment? I decided to send thank-you cards a few days after each interview, and this gesture was readily acknowledged by women I did see again. Women offered many thanks for the time I had spent with them, both at the time of interview and if I happened to see them again at a support group or by chance.

Whilst the initial method of inquiry was to be interviews alone, I quickly felt the need to read these women's stories against the broader context of breast cancer culture. In order to 'see' this larger framework I immersed myself in the breast cancer community, attending support groups, fundraising events, advocacy group meetings, hospital programs, frequently visiting breast cancer websites, reading any text or video-based information that was given to women who were diagnosed, reading breast cancer organization newsletters, and attending or informing myself about any relevant conferences.

As I go on to show, all of these sites of analysis enable important links to be established between the microparticulars found in interview accounts and macrocultural structures.[6] At all of these 'sites of practice' discourses are constructed which situate women, bodies and health as particular things in particular frameworks of meaning.[7]

Getting interviews participants

In order to recruit women to my study I placed short advertisements in three Australian breast cancer support network newsletters: Bosom Buddies (ACT), Breast Cancer Action Group (Victoria) and The Beacon (newsletter of the Breast Cancer Network Australia). These newsletters reach over 1000 women across Victoria, the ACT and NSW. In addition, I attended the ACT Cancer Society Breast Cancer Support Group and a Bosom Buddies General Meeting, where I handed out brief summaries of my research with a slip at the bottom where women could fill out their name and phone number and the best time for me to call. I received about 50 responses initially and continued to receive enquiries via phone calls and emails for about six months following the initial advertisements. Of these 50, 30 women were interviewed, selected basically depending on the accessibility to their house. For example, several women responded from the Northern Territory, Northern NSW and Queensland; however, it was impossible for me to travel to do these interviews. Phone interviews were an option but I decided against this because of the number of responses I had received already and realizing the limitations of my thesis.

In addition to obtaining participants via advertisements and attending Breast Cancer groups, I made contact with women by snowball sampling. Quite often after I had interviewed someone they would tell me of a friend who had breast cancer who was interested in my research or who they thought would be a good person to interview. In these cases I sent information to these women about my research and left it up to them to contact me to avoid pressure.

Once I had been contacted by the interested respondent, I chatted with them over the phone answering any questions about my research interests and aims, and what would be required of them in the interview. This discussion usually lasted about 10–20 minutes and we would arrange a suitable time for me to do the interview.

Research setting

The majority of the interviews were carried out in participants' homes. We usually sat at the kitchen table or in the lounge room – somewhere that allowed me to place my tape recorder easily. Three of the interviews were carried out in my university office, three were carried out at participants' workplaces. One interview was conducted at my home, as the woman felt uncomfortable doing it in her own home where her family was around. The setting for the interview was always chosen by the participant, usually as the most convenient or comfortable place for them.

The interview

The interview would usually begin about 10–20 minutes after my arrival. General discussion always preceded the interview – how long she had lived at her particular house, or information about her children or family.

They all asked me general information about where I had come from and where I lived. Conversation was always sparked by my engagement ring and quite often discussion about the particulars of my upcoming wedding bridged the gap between stranger and friend. Over a cup of tea we would get to know each other briefly before I would ask her to describe when she first found out she had breast cancer. Indeed the success of the research depended upon my being able to form relationships with the participants.

All of the women readily agreed to have their interviews tape recorded. However, conversation often flowed more freely once the tape recorder was turned off, as the participant offered information about things she thought irrelevant to my research, for example details of relationship breakups or hassles at work. I never felt that the participant was holding anything back in the interview; on the contrary, I was surprised by the openness, honesty and explicitness of detail these women shared with me. Often in the conversation the participant would preface what she was saying with 'I don't think this is what you want' or 'this is probably irrelevant, but . . .'. I always encouraged her to keep going by saying that whatever she thought was relevant, was relevant to her experience and therefore relevant for my purposes, and even if it did not seem outwardly 'what I wanted' it was often crucial to her contextualization of her story and her life.

Over the course of my interviews I never became de-sensitized to a woman crying or telling me horrific tales of surgery or fears of dying. I was always affected by the interview, by some more than others, but always with a feeling that something *very real* had taken place. What I took away from the interview was rich both for my purposes of data and analysis and for me as a person. Over and over again women said how since being diagnosed with cancer they did not worry about the little things in life – the house being dirty or denting the car, these were small matters in the scheme of things. Facing death had made them 'realize what priorities were', and that life and relationships were what mattered. I found myself repeating their words when arguing with my fiancé, wanting to put things into perspective and suggesting that there were bigger and more important things in life than dirty dishes or misspent money.

Involvement, detachment and responsibility

As much as I was moved by these interviews I was also frustrated and felt quite helpless. I often thought that I had not 'given back' what had been given to me in the process of the interview. I wished I could offer good advice and often felt I was more an ill-equipped counsellor than a learning researcher. Still it was impossible not to offer gentle advice, reaffirm feelings of worth or dismiss feelings of worthlessness or abnormality. Never was I more acutely aware of this than during my interview with Rita. Divorced and living alone, Rita, 56, was a social worker who had retired due to her multiple ill-health conditions, and felt she had been emotionally abandoned by her family. She had a lumpectomy seven years prior to our meeting and had subsequent treatment. Since then she had had four other lumps removed all of which had been found to be benign. The interview began as I walked through the door, and lasted about four hours. Rita told me a very sad story about her life, with breast cancer being another in a long line of unfortunate experiences. At the end of her life story narrative Rita said that she had decided to end her life and that she had been feeling suicidal since her last lumpectomy three months before. In three hours of interview I had not said a word, except for nods and exclamations. After she revealed her suicidal feelings, I found myself racing to think of the right thing to say. My emotions were mixed, stemming from growing up in a family that has been affected by suicide to understanding her rationale after a life of abuse, ill-health and abandonment, to desperation at wanting her to see that she was an intelligent, strong and amazing woman who had so much to live for.

In such a situation it seemed inadequate to hand her a card with the number of a support group on it, as I had outlined I would do in my ethics form. As a researcher I knew, theoretically, my 'job' was to listen. I should acknowledge that I was a part of the interview as much as the participant, but not to give advice as such, neither medical nor personal. But as a woman, as a person, I did have a responsibility here. We talked through her strengths and how she could use these strengths, and I openly told her of my concern at her thoughts of suicide. We slowly moved on to topics of her delight at her new grandchild and she showed me photos of him and shared some of the funny stories of him when he visited. Before I left we agreed I would call her in a few days and I would give some other telephone numbers of people she could speak to over the phone and get advice. I hopped in the car, drove about two blocks away, then pulled over shaken and crying. What was my responsibility? I phoned her later that day urging her to call Lifeline and with the promise of calling her again. I did phone a couple of times and only got her answering machine, I left various numbers for her to call. About one week later Rita phoned me to say 'thank you'. She told me that she felt much better after our morning together, saying that all she had needed was for someone to listen to her and take her seriously.

This highlighted for me the fact that I had not been useless and in fact in all of my interviews I was instrumental in giving permission to women to talk openly about their lives in a very personal and honest way. This permission was given through body language, in facial expressions, nods of reassurance, laughter, smiling, frowning at tales of mistreatment or being made feel stupid by doctors or family. In addition it was important to be a compassionate listener, allowing the participant to talk freely without cutting her off, in letting her story take whatever path she wanted it to take, and encouraging her to share as much or as little as she wanted about particular topics. It was important to recognize when she felt uncomfortable but wanted to keep talking through it, or uncomfortable and wanted to stop.

I attended one funeral during my interviewing process. I had interviewed Diane, 59, about a month prior to her death. She had been diagnosed with advanced breast cancer and spoke with me at length about her experience of breast cancer and her fears of dying. When I heard of the news that she had passed away I was unsure about the appropriateness of my attending the funeral service. I had met this woman on a number of occasions, first during the interview and twice since then at support group meetings. I had spent a morning with Diane and her husband, talking in depth about her cancer, her coping mechanisms, her sexuality and identity and her relationship with her husband.

I spent a couple of days wondering whether I should go to the funeral. Was I a friend or would I be intruding? My dilemma was solved when I received an email from Diane's husband informing me of the details of the funeral service. I felt welcomed and did not think about it again. Attending Diane's funeral had a significant impact on how I felt about my research. I knew that breast cancer was a life threatening illness, however, I do not think the reality of that struck me until the service. I sat amongst a large group of women who I had interviewed and they held my hands throughout. Although an outsider I felt welcomed into their lives.

In a couple of instances the woman's husband sat with her during our interview, usually offering tid bits of information, or corrections on details of her treatment. Although I am sure their presence shaped the form of interview in some way it never seemed to restrict the participant in her answers or descriptions.

Debriefing

After the tape recorder was turned off and I had signalled the end of the interview there was a debriefing period of 30 minutes to up to an hour or more. During this time we talked about more general issues again, and if the participant had become upset during the interview I stayed until she was no longer distressed and we were talking and laughing about the positives of her experience with breast cancer, or matters altogether different. On a number of occasions I was offered lunch or dinner at the end of the interview, which sometimes I took up, depending on my own time restrictions. This debriefing was a crucial part of the interview, for both the participant and myself. For me, these interviews were emotionally exhausting, some more so than others; and for the participant, issues were discussed that she had perhaps not articulated before, or not in quite a long time. In all but a couple of my 30 interviews the participant cried at some time. I carried out at most two interviews per day, making sure I had plenty of time after each one to debrief.

Presentation of the self as researcher

According to Shaffir *et al.*:

> The intensity of the fieldwork process is typically accompanied by a psychological anxiety resulting in a continuous presentation and management of the self when in the presence of those studied. (1980: 4)

'Psychological anxiety' is perhaps too strong a phrase to attribute to my own feelings while conducting the fieldwork; however, I did experience a certain amount of self-consciousness. The dilemma of what to wear to the interview is one that researchers have noted before,[8] trying to find the right mix of casual and unintimidating with smart and professional. One thing that struck me when I first started interviewing was how conscious I was of my own breasts. I felt self-conscious in two ways. First I was aware of how they were presented in the actual interview. I tried to find clothes that were not tight or revealing, nothing that would emphasize my chest at all. In articulating this it seems quite ridiculous, but the inappropriateness I felt about it at the time was significant. While talking with women about the grief they felt over the loss of their own breasts, I did not want to be emphasizing my own. Throughout the interview I felt self-conscious, relaxing my posture so as to not accentuate my bust. Secondly, I became aware of them in terms of constantly checking for lumps. I had a sense that everyone I knew had breast cancer and I became obsessive in self-examination. I became more aware of what this part of my body meant to me and what it would mean if they were not there. In the latter part of writing up my doctorate I became pregnant and gave birth to my first child. The acute awareness of my ever increasing bust and then breastfeeding grounded some of the words I had been hearing from participants about attachment to breasts through nurturing their children. I was able to acknowledge and understand the bond women had described to me.

Demographics of interview participants

In this study, 30 women were interviewed, all of which were tape recorded. Of these, 26 were able to be successfully transcribed, but in four only field notes were used due to technical difficulties with recordings. From these four no quotes are used in this book.

The number of women chosen for this study was based on reaching a point of saturation during the interviewing process. I was unsure of how many women I would need and decided to do as many interviews as possible until I found themes started to be repeated and I was gaining nothing new from subsequent interviews. Furthermore, although each interview provided its own valuable and individual insight, after 30, I found I was emotionally exhausted from the process and the size of the practical task of transcribing was becoming apparent.

Of the women interviewed, 25 were from the ACT, including Queanbeyan and Jerrabomberra (NSW suburbs just outside Canberra), four were from Melbourne, Victoria and one was from Deniliquin, in country NSW. These women were at differing stages in their treatment for breast cancer. Five were going through treatment (chemotherapy) at the time of interview, one for advanced breast cancer (for further details, see Table 1.1a). Four women I spoke to had had breast cancer twice. Of these two had recurrences within two years of initial diagnosis, one had a recurrence seven years after initial diagnosis and the other after 10 years. Treatment for cancer varied from chemotherapy alone, radiotherapy, a mixture of both or surgery without other treatment, and two had sought alternative therapies from naturopaths and homeopaths. A number also mentioned being on Tamoxifen after chemotherapy and radiotherapy had ceased.

Some women had experienced a lumpectomy, subsequent mastectomy and then having the second breast removed. Although only four had reconstructions a number were currently seeing surgeons with a view of having reconstruction done in the near future. Occupations fell broadly into the white collar worker category: school teachers, nurses, public servants, social workers, bank manager, university staff, private family business, lab technician and secretary. The majority were married with children (Table 1.1b), educated with either a higher degree or further

Table 1.1a Summary information about interview participants: Age and surgery

Age at time of interview		Age at time of diagnosis		Time from diagnosis and treatment at interview (years)		Extent of surgery			
Range	Mean	Range	Mean	Range	Mean	Lumpectomy or partial mastectomy only	Unilateral mastectomy	Bilateral mastectomy	Reconstruction
33–64	52	32–63	47	Present–14	7	12	10	8	4

Table 1.1b Summary information about interview participants: Marital and maternal status

Married with children	Married without children	Divorced	Widowed	Never married
18	5	5	1	1

training and all were English speaking, white, heterosexual and middle-class women.

Breast cancer incidence

Breast cancer is a significant health problem in the industrialized Western world, where it is the most common form of cancer among women in North America, Australia and almost all of Europe. It is estimated that each year the disease is diagnosed in over one million women world-wide and is the cause of death in over 400,000 women.[9] The incidence of the disease is increasing, in both industrialized and developing countries. In the United States, for example, the incidence rate for breast cancer has increased steadily by about 1–2 per cent per year since 1960.[10]

Data from Australia, the United States and the United Kingdom all suggest that there has been a substantial reduction in breast cancer mortality in recent years,[11] a decrease that suggests it is due to improvements in the way breast cancer has been diagnosed and treated. However, at present in both the United States and the United Kingdom 1 in 9 women are expected to be diagnosed with breast cancer before the age of 75 and 1 in 11 women in Australia. The incidence rate for breast cancer is more than three times that of any other cancer in females and the mortality rate is 60 per cent higher than that of lung cancer, the second most common cause of cancer death in females.[12]

Age is the most recognized risk factor for breast cancer, and incidence increases with age. It is believed that women of high socio-economic status are at greater risk of breast cancer than women of low socio-economic status, perhaps because of differences in reproductive history, lifestyle factors and proportionally more well-educated women attending mammography screening. In addition the risk of breast cancer is doubled among women with a first-degree relative diagnosed with breast cancer before the age of 40 years.[13]

It is these commonly flagged statistics that capture the attention of women, medical professionals, policy makers and prosthetics manufacturers.

Breast cancer surgery

Almost every form of breast cancer will involve some surgery. Surgical management may begin with the biopsy of a lump detected by the woman herself, her partner, her doctor or a mammogram or other type of screening. Although there are various forms of biopsies, they generally involve the removal of at least a number of the suspect cells, and at most the removal of the entire lump.

In the past the surgical management of breast cancer involved only one operation, the Halstead Radical Mastectomy, which required the removal of the entire breast and surrounding tissues and muscle. In recent years this approach has been replaced by several less radical options, namely partial mastectomy or lumpectomy, quadrantectomy – involving the removal of a large section of the breast – and total mastectomy, which unlike its predecessor does not usually involve removal of pectoral muscles. In all cases lymph nodes may be taken. Depending on the location of the cancerous tissue, the nipple may not be removed, even if all other breast tissue is excised. There can be considerable nerve damage and a loss of some or all sensitivity to the surrounding tissue. In any case, the woman's body is cut and scarred, and looks and feels different to what it did prior to the surgery.

Nearly half of breast cancer patients will lose an entire breast,[14] a proportion that has decreased since 1986 when most (78%) breast cancer operations were mastectomies. This is due to the increase of breast-conserving surgery, where surgeons opt to take only the cancerous tissue and usually some surrounding tissue from the breast in hope that it has not spread further. Studies of patterns of surgical management of breast cancer show that choices by surgeons regarding extent of surgery are based on practical as well as cosmetic outcomes. For example, the tendency for rural women to undergo mastectomy rather than breast-conserving surgery may reflect the lack of access to post-operative radio-therapy.[15] It has also been argued, however, that treatment is mainly dependent on surgeons' individual preferences.[16]

Women are commonly offered two methods of restoring breast shape following breast loss: prosthesis or surgical reconstruction.

Prostheses

A prosthesis, or breast form, is a detachable object that sits inside a bra or adheres to the skin to create a breast shape. Usually made from silicone or foam, prostheses come in a range of differing sizes, weights and shapes and can be tailored for use during different activities. Swimming prostheses, for example, are lightweight and waterproof making them less likely to 'pop' out of bathers.

When they are in hospital recovering from surgery, most women are offered 'temporary' cotton wool prostheses meant for use until the woman is able to get to a professional prosthesis fitter. Costing between

Aus$200 and Aus$400, prostheses last only a couple of years, requiring women to continually purchase new ones. If a woman wants to restore breast shape but seeks an alternative to prostheses, various methods of surgical reconstruction are available.

Reconstruction

Through improved surgical techniques over the past 100 years, reconstructive breast surgery has become less invasive and enabled better cosmetic results.[17] In Australia, reconstruction is the choice of 20 per cent of all women who have had a breast amputated. In the United States and United Kingdom it is a more common choice with up to 50 per cent of women requesting reconstruction. According to the American Society of Plastic Surgeons (ASPS) breast reconstruction after mastectomy rose 180 per cent from 1992 to 1999 due to increased insurance coverage and education.

Most reconstructions are delayed, that is, conducted as a second operation after the patient has recovered from her mastectomy.[18] Alternatively, women may choose an immediate reconstruction whereby the breast is reconstructed at the same time as mastectomy. Women therefore wake up having lost their original breast but with another in its place.

Breast reconstruction is not just an operation, rather as one surgeon informed me, it is a programme. What follows the decision to have surgery is a cavalcade of decisions regarding type of surgery, size and shape of new breast/s, additional surgery to the natural breast to lift, fill out or reduce it and the type of nipple restoration. There are two main techniques of reconstruction, either insertion of an implant of some kind or a type of 'flap' reconstruction requiring a woman's own muscle and skin from the back, abdomen or hip being transplanted to the chest to form the reconstructed breast.

The complexity of women's dealings with breast cancer and surgery and breast restoration has inspired much research. This book examines the production of breast cancer knowledge, the renegotiation of identity during and after a breast cancer crisis, the disconnection of body and self that may occur as a result of cancer treatment and breast loss, and draws attention to what is left unsaid about the post-surgical body. These themes have been identified and explored by various scholars through a variety of theoretical and methodological approaches.

Approaches to breast cancer and the post-surgical body

There are a number of different frameworks, or ways in which people have talked about the post-surgical body in the past. These range from biomedical and scientific analyses to anthropological, sociological and psychosocial analyses, and health promotion literature and autobiographical accounts.

While reading this literature I asked many questions: Who or what was the subject in the research? Was it the woman with breast cancer or was it a specific surgical technique that was the focus? Who was it being written for? An audience of academics, women with an interest in breast cancer or perhaps medical specialists? How were women's experiences represented in the text? How did the authors legitimate their research and how then did they assert their authority on the subject? Finally, what was not asked by the researchers? What do these silences reveal?

Medical knowledge has been seen as the benevolent application of objective knowledge through scientific methods. Traditionally, medical knowledge is conflated with truth and objectivity and as such stands at an untouchable and unquestionable distance. The medical approach to studying breast cancer and mastectomy is based on dominant biomedical knowledge that claims to be based on a purely objective rationale. Biomedical knowledge both derives from and aligns with science in order to bolster its legitimacy.

Scientific literature on breast cancer tends to focus upon the breast as an anatomical structure, independent of the woman attached or the surgical technique used to treat or remove the breast. The audience is almost entirely other medical specialists. Women's experiences are represented either through the author's generalizations, that is, 'most women want their breasts reconstructed', or as a statistic, that is, '80 per cent of women are happy with the result'. Medical literature is legitimated by the authors clinical training or references to a 'controlled' trial and also in the assumption that women will want to 'get back to normal', that is, regain two breasts. The text is thus able to assert its authority using technical language and in distancing itself from the subject by writing in the third person.

The questions such studies ask for example are as follows: What are the surgical management options available? How many days after surgery should the patient be discharged? What is the failure rate of a particular surgical technique? What types of reconstructions or prostheses are available for a woman post-mastectomy?

Traditionally, social research into the way that women make sense of cancer in general and breast cancer specifically has been from within medical disciplines and concerned with issues of decision making, coping mechanisms, and risk assessment and management. While the majority of this research has done much to further our understanding of some of the parameters of women's experiences of breast cancer, most use quantitative measures of women's moods, attitudes, coping behaviours and quality of life and have been criticized for their limited ability to capture the depth and complexity of women's perceptions and experiences.[19] In general, by relying on numerical ratings, this type of research presents women with an already defined framework of meaning, and measures how women fit within this framework.[20]

There has been an increase in qualitative research that legitimates women's voices and acknowledges women as 'experts' over their own lives. Such studies have looked at how life experiences and belief systems influence the way women interpret, confront and examine the meanings of health.[21] Although much has been written on breast cancer and the effect of the disease on women's bodies, until the time of writing there has been little that stems from feminist and sociological perspectives. This book has been largely informed by the academic and personal insights of Anne Kasper (1994, 1995), Susan Ferguson (2000, with Kasper 2000), Mira Crouch and Heather McKenzie (2000), Dorothy Broom (2001), Sue Wilkinson (1998, 2000, 2001, with Kitzinger 1994, 2000) and Lenore Manderson (1999) all of whom have made important contributions to the study of breast cancer in general, and the mastectomized body and breast restoration in particular.

My analysis touches on and extends themes that have been identified and explored by these scholars. For example, I argue that identity and breast loss are linked[22] and I examine the discursive and material practices which reproduce a woman's post-surgical self and body in potentially damaging ways. I explore the influence that the medical profession and prosthetic manufacturers have in contributing to women's decision making regarding breast restoration,[23] making more explicit the active role women play in reproducing aesthetic norms. I pay attention to the ways women are situated as at risk of revealing the truth about their mastectomized bodies[24] identifying specific sites where this is perpetuated. A constant theme in this book is the link between *looking* and *feeling* well[25] and the limited options women are given to deal with their post-surgical bodies.[26] I examine the material-semiotic practices of the post-surgical body: how women *do* their bodies in everyday existence. I want to bring the mastectomized body into focus, revealing the personal and cultural narratives of this body and the implications for a woman's self.

Femininity, gender and embodiment

The lived experience of both *being* a body and *having* a body is central to the sociology of health and illness. When illness occurs, aspects of the body that were previously taken for granted are brought into focus. As medical anthropologist Byron Good notes, for the person who is experiencing illness or pain, 'the body is not simply a physical object or physiological state but an essential part of the self' (1994: 116).

This study seeks to understand how women who have undergone a mastectomy experience their altered bodies. Focusing on issues such as stigma and embarrassment, Goffman provides an understanding of how the body mediates between social-identity and self-identity. In his work *The Presentation of Self in Everyday Life* (1956), he examined how people tactically present themselves in ways to counter socially undesirable or negative experiences. He argues that self-presentations or 'performances' are socially constructed for public audiences to maintain social identities. In doing so, he is able to highlight the important role of human emotions, feelings and sentiments and the 'circuits of selfhood' they involve.

A key contribution of this book lies in the examination of the relationship between this experience of embodiment and breast cancer culture. For Goffman, successful passage through public space is both a practical problem and a skilful accomplishment for the human agent, involving specific social roles and rituals which facilitate this passage and 'repair' disruptions to the micropublic order of social interaction. As I go on to show, the mastectomized body presents a disruption to both a social and a self-identity.

A major theme of this book is the effort required by mastectomized women to come to terms with, conceal, and/or accept their post-surgical body. Tensions between a previously 'whole' self and a new, altered self emerge when faced with discourse that projects identity as strongly connected with the essence of womanhood (that essence being a femininity defined by breasts). To examine women's experiences of breast cancer thus requires more than simply treating them as the 'human agents' Goffman describes. In addition, exploration of the lived body needs to take account of the particular *gendered* modalities, structures and conditions of our embodied being-in-the-world.[27]

This challenge is taken up by Young (1990), for instance, in her classic phenomenological study *Throwing like a girl*. Young suggests that women's social *training* makes them less equipped to act in space (for example, when catching a ball) and that women are more aware of themselves as *objects* (i.e., through the objectifying male gaze). She argues that women, as lived bodies, are not 'open' and 'unambiguous transcendences' that move out to 'master a world that belongs to us, a world constituted by our own intentions and projects'. Rather, they are 'physically handicapped' in a 'sexist society'.[28]

Following breast cancer surgery, and the objectifying process of breast cancer treatment, many women are expected to feel 'physically handicapped' not only because of a patriarchal society which exults in breasts, but also because in the world of breast cancer culture regaining symmetrical breastedness is taken as one and the same as regaining what is feminine. Women's one-breasted bodies are cast as 'other' against a sometimes unattainable and unnecessary 'norm'.

What it is to be 'feminine' has been addressed by Judith Butler in her work on gender as a performance. Butler (1990, 1993) attempts to argue that the 'sexed' body is simultaneously biology and culture, materiality and inscription. In other words, it is an ideal construct that is forcibly materialized through time: 'It is not a simple fact or static condition of the body, but a process whereby regulatory norms materialize sex...through a forcible reiteration of those norms'.[29] Seen in these terms 'sex' is not simply what one has, or what one is, rather it is something that is repeatedly performed into existence in everyday gestures. In this thesis, the body is not only something which is performed, it is regarded as a site of social, political, cultural and geographical inscription.[30]

Language as discourse

The humanities and social sciences have experienced a growing interest in language and discourse in the past three decades. This 'linguistic turn' has seen a 'preoccupation with recognising and understanding the role of language in constituting and maintaining social order and notions of reality'.[31] Discourse and the reality to which it pertains are no longer seen as separate things, rather discourse is seen as constitutive of what counts as reality. In this way discourses are patterns of words, figures of speech, concepts, values and symbols, all of which provide a means of 'making sense' of an object, person, social group or event.[32]

The works of Emily Martin (1987) and Susan Sontag (1978, 1989) draw attention to the importance of language in the construction of women's bodies in medicine. Emily Martin (1987) uses the deconstruction of medical metaphors as a theoretical tool to illustrate how such tropes remove our bodily functions from reality, further fragmenting women's experience of body and self. Similarly, Sontag (1978) highlights the impact of the use of military metaphors when talking about cancer as they discursively produce illness as a 'battle' to be won and the cancer 'invading' and trying to 'conquer' the body. Language is performative and brings certain forms of knowledge and action into being.

Lupton (1994a) argues that practices constitute and reinforce existing discourses, and vice versa. Language is therefore self-performative, it *does* the object, person and so on in a particular way and produces certain understandings and meanings. This move towards examining the practices of discursive production has important implications for the examination of narratives of illness so often used in the sociology of health and medicine.

In *Teratologies: A Cultural Study of Cancer* Jackie Stacey argues, 'illnesses become narratives very quickly' (1997: 5), as the past is transformed into narrative coherence. Stacey focuses attention on the importance of language as constructing a person's illness and self in particular ways. Thus the stories that people tell *about* their illness trajectory are embedded in historical, political and cultural settings, shaped usually unknowingly by social structures, relations of power and the nature of the social practices in which they are engaged. Discourses are therefore not just 'words'; they are material-semiotic practices through which objects of attention and knowing subjects are both constituted.[33] People therefore *do* the 'object of attention' in giving their narrative, and the post-surgical body is constructed and performed in the telling of their stories.

Performing the body

Within science and technology studies there has been a significant shift towards looking at practices, in attending to the *doing*. Interactionist Science Studies (ISS) looks at the doing of scientific work; at how it is situated and 'done in particular spaces, times and locations, with particular material practices'.[34] Fundamental to ISS is the dissolution of the distinction between knowledge and practice. It is through practices and interaction that knowledge is generated. ISS talks about these material practices as being constructed by the various participants in specific locations, as being co-constructed, or 'mutually articulated'[35] through interactions among the given elements in the situation. Through a framework that attends not only to subjects, but to objects, we can begin to unravel the processes in action to understand how knowledge is produced. This shift to paying attention to the material suggests that discourse thought of as words is closely mixed in with practices. Indeed words and things are ordered in practice.

Breast cancer and the post-surgical body are not something we *have* and talk *about*, rather they are *performed*. The post-surgical body is *done* in particular ways and is therefore not a singular entity but multiple. Through a performative lens, the post-surgical body can be seen as existing not as one, but many; as performed in a variety of ways.[36]

Similarly, gender is not something we essentially have, rather it is something that we *do*.[37] This *doing* of gender is thus located in the everyday gestures and movements that constitute the illusion of an abiding gendered self. Butler (1990) argues that the 'reality' of gender is created through sustained social performances.

Scholars of narrative analysis such as Susan Sontag, Arthur Frank and Arthur Kleinman analyse stories and their meaning, and how stories structure experience retrospectively. The lived body is thus something that is embodied through cultural discourse and can be analysed by paying attention to the linguistic. Alternatively, Judith Butler and Annemarie Mol are not interested in stories and their meaning, they suggest things such as gender are performances, not stable or fixed, but multiple and ever changing. In this text, I want to treat language as a vital part of that performance, whether it is how and what is spoken about in interviews, or what is written in information given to women during breast cancer treatment. Language, most often talking, is a central part of women's recovery from breast cancer. It is the focal point of most support group programs and advocacy group meetings and it plays a crucial role in the way women's experiences are projected. So too is the physicality of their body during this, for example, wearing a prosthesis or not. To me, language is a central tenet of the performativity thesis, not an alternative.

One could argue that the performativity thesis is an epistemological debate about the importance of not taking 'things' for granted. Typically performativity refers to specific ways of *doing* that does not necessarily include the linguistic. By extension, this thesis demonstrates that by treating language as a major component of the way women manage their post surgical body, the experience of mastectomy is unpacked to reveal the complexity of embodiment (an epistemological point) *and* the implications this has on a pragmatic level. Paying attention to how a woman displays, hides, relates to or co-exists with her changed body and its subsequent appendages (prostheses, implants) reveals much about the impact breast surgery has on her day-to-day life, whether it be answering the door, giving someone a hug or playing sport. Similarly, focusing on the ways women who have had breast surgery are marketed, represented, advised and spoken about and to impacts the way a woman may dress, the post-operative path she may take (restoration or not), her approach to her relationships and her self perception.

Many women with breast cancer articulate a loss of femininity when their breasts are removed. Women feel they no longer identify as 'complete' or 'whole'. The question arises: Did their breasts define their femininity prior to their removal? Indeed women in this study describe only worrying about them when they are threatened or taken away. This is perhaps because femininity is an essence that we assume is biologically expressed. Through a performative lens femininity is performed into existence. The question then is how do mastectomized women do that with the new materialities of the post-surgical body?

This book addresses issues of language, materiality and performativity through analyses of women's stories of breast cancer and surgery, their practices and the institutions of breast cancer.

Book structure

Chapter 2 explores women's narratives as a point of reflexivity where experience and self converge. I ask *how* women are identifying and positioning themselves in these stories, and what the implications are when they identify themselves in these ways. I pay close attention to the accounts of three women and explore four main themes: (1) the construction of breast cancer knowledge; (2) the renegotiation of identity during and after breast cancer and surgery; (3) the disconnection of body and self and (4) silences of the post-surgical body. These themes are explored in depth in subsequent chapters and provide the theoretical underpinnings of this book. Chapter 2 aims to ground these themes within whole accounts. In the chapter, I argue that women draw on different discourses to articulate their illness experience but give similar references to broader cultural narratives of the body. While Nell, Rita and Jacqui all draw from readily available scripts to discuss their illness, no such scripts exist for talking about their post-surgical bodies. The post-surgical body is situated as a site of ambiguity and anxiety as women draw from a prefigured discourse of the mastectomized body which positions it in negative terms. As a result tensions emerge between the body and the self as these women try to fit their experiences within this frame.

Chapter 3 examines how mainstream breast cancer culture reproduces these narratives of the post-surgical body. This chapter is concerned with the construction of meanings of the post-surgical body within the breast cancer movement and its subsequent influence on a woman's illness experience. I ask how this culture contributes to the framing of the post-surgical body. I argue that mainstream breast cancer culture mobilizes a specific breast cancer identity which promotes aesthetic hegemony and frames the mastectomized body as unfeminine, abnormal and desexualized. Breast cancer culture promotes a discourse which assumes all women will want to restore their breasts thus ensuring a reinstatement of femininity, normalcy and acceptance into society. In addition a 'keep it in the closet' ideology is perpetuated that provides no space for women to think about alternatives to breast prostheses or reconstruction. This secrecy is overcompensated for by a very public feminine themed advocacy, which further mobilizes the mastectomized body as something to be embarrassed about and kept hidden. I argue that individual and public challenges to these norms could begin to destabilize such stereotypes and allow women more freedom of choice when coming to terms with their changed bodies.

In Chapter 4, I examine the commodification of the post-surgical body by prosthesis companies, the medical profession and cancer organizations. All three provide powerful discourses that present the post-surgical body as incomplete and abnormal in the absence of two breasts. Furthermore, a failure to restore the body to its pre-cancer appearance is viewed as an incomplete recovery. I examine the mobilization of the prosthesis as a nexus between body and self. Recovering from a breast cancer crisis is thus linked with restoring breast shape and conforming to dominant notions of femininity. But *how* are these tropes, which situate women's post-surgical bodies as incomplete and lacking femininity and sexuality produced? How is the post-surgical body defined and constituted? I examine the meanings women attribute to their mastectomy and the ways they successfully and unsuccessfully attempt to integrate the prosthesis into their self and daily life. I go on to explore how issues of body image are linked to femininity and identity in information booklets given to women during their illness. I show how these texts situate emotional and physical recovery as intricately linked to restoring breast shape. I explore the powerful influence of prostheses manufacturers who tie traditional notions of how the female body should look and act with recovery from a breast cancer crisis. Using themes of science and technology, liberation and femininity, and metaphors of being 'complete' and 'natural', advertisements for prostheses not only sell the usefulness of their devices but market certain understandings and meanings of the post-surgical body. Finally, by examining the daily practices required of wearing prostheses discrepancies emerge as the prosthesis as a nexus between body and self is revealed to be unstable.

An analysis of breast reconstruction in Chapter 5 considers the construction of choice for women to deal with their self and body after a mastectomy. In this chapter, I ask how does breast reconstruction figure in the remaking of self following mastectomy? For women who have a breast amputated, the option of breast reconstruction constructs a sense of hope of regaining lost femininity, sexuality and normalcy.

In conclusion I draw out the implications of the current status of the mastectomized body. I ask what can be done to widen the discursive depictions of the mastectomized body and include a possibility for refusal of breast restoration. I argue that breast reconstruction is seen to be not only aesthetically desirable, but is also seen as a woman's post-mastectomy journey back to femininity and identity.

2
Narratives of the Self

Introduction: Narrative analysis

The use of narrative analysis in health research has attracted increased attention in recent years with patient's narratives giving voice to suffering in a way that traditionally lies outside the domain of biomedicine.[1] As a methodological tool, illness narratives have been used in varying ways, with varying depths of analysis. I have identified four broad ways that researchers use illness narratives to explore the world of 'biomedical reality, illness experience and its social and cultural underpinnings'.[2]

First, research has focused on the importance of storytelling to deal with a traumatic event.[3] At this level, analysis of illness narratives can identify and explore themes and issues of importance for the patient and/or carer.[4] However, such studies have been criticized for tending to assume a certain 'transparency' with regard to the illness story, seeing it as an '(in)authentic reflection of the individual's experience, often constructed in opposition to the largely objectifying and deindividualizing "voice" of medical technology'.[5]

Secondly, narratives are used to ascertain attitudes and belief systems, and how such beliefs influence opinions, interactions and meaning making.[6] Narratives are thus used to build conceptual frameworks where beliefs, interpretation, understanding, agency and subjective well-being intersect.

Thirdly, a growing number of researchers have extended the use of illness narratives to look at how the narrative fits into broader cultural narratives and to what extent these cultural narratives construct events.[7] Such research illuminates how practices and understandings are embedded within and reproduced by the larger narrative and how shared understandings shape the interpretation and construction of individual experience.

Lastly, authors analyse narrative structure, identifying varying forms that storytelling may take.[8] Frank classifies illness narratives in accordance with three 'storylines': 'restitution', 'chaos' and 'quest', which he identifies as typifying the understanding of illness, its course and process and its relation to a person's own life.[9] The implications of such predetermined scripts mean that patients are often pressured to take up narratives that cast them outside the discourse of everyday life, as either passive victims or courageous heroes.[10] Alternatively, Hyden (1997) suggests a typology that is based on the formal aspects of illness narratives, namely the relationship between narrator, narrative and illness. He suggests three *types* of illness narratives: illness *as* narrative, narrative *about* illness and narrative *as* illness. Hyden's typology is not based on a limited set of narrative genres, as is the case with Frank. Instead he suggests there is a variety of types of narratives with widely divergent functions.

Less prolific in the literature on narratives is the exploration of the connections between experiential accounts and the wider currency that such accounts take on when viewed in light of the discourses that privilege or allow such narratives. In addition, the relationship between experience and the context of illness is less often studied, despite its importance for demonstrating the pragmatic aspects of the current contributions of medical anthropology and sociology.[11] This context identifies how the patient's experience takes shape and acquires meaning through such aspects as historical and cultural frameworks in which, for example, breast cancer imagery has been constructed.[12] Breast cancer is therefore 'not just a personal process but rather an experience filtered through the meanings constructed by the social context'.[13] Consequently, language is a major locus of knowledge, personifying causes and giving coherence to illness.[14]

The way that stories are embedded in 'grand narratives' and the tropes that act to reproduce them are seldom explored in depth, and as such the full potential of narrative analysis is perhaps not realized. Frank (1998) has gone some way to highlight the importance of looking beyond the importance of the 'story', illuminating the 'manufacturing process' that goes into the production of stories of self and illness, looking, for example, at how power is implicated in such stories.

Breast cancer, like other illnesses, disrupts the person's life as it was known previously. Life is thrown into chaos as the patient attempts to make sense of and situate herself amongst all that is happening. In a sense we make order out of chaos by the accounts we construct of ourselves. Saillant argues that explanations of illness 'from the patient's point of view' give rise to a symbolization process which, in turn, allows the experience to be situated within a whole (1990: 97). This 'whole' is both physical and emotional and gives meaning and coherence to illness and survival.

When talking with women about their experience of breast cancer and breast surgery what they emphasized, what they left out, their words and phrases and the relationship of those words and phrases to their story, all indicate a positioning of the self. This positioning highlights ways in which they identify themselves and others in their own narrative. As Hyden suggests 'the narrative's importance lies in its being one of the main forms through which we perceive, experience, and judge our actions and the course and value of our lives' (1997: 49).

Framing of narrative

Both Hyden (1997) and Frank (1995) give detailed typologies of illness narratives, suggesting that narratives take quite specific forms. In my interviews I found that women's narratives constituted a medical history and a personal life history. The narratives were overlapping and sometimes contradictory. Whilst it is important to locate the tropes and discourses that allow or 'privilege' their individual narratives, it is also significant to identify what is not said or so easily articulated.

The narrative is a point of reflexivity where experience and self converge. According to Giddens (1990, 1991) this is a way to transcend the dualism between biomedical and social constructions of the body. In telling their stories women are able to make sense of what they are experiencing. My question is *how* are women identifying and positioning themselves in these narratives, and what are the implications when they identify themselves in these ways?

In what follows I examine three case studies, chosen because they represent the diversity of experience of my interview participants and also because they contain many themes that were common in all interviews. Each woman is at a different stage in her illness experience. Nell, 58, has a family history of breast cancer. She was diagnosed four years ago and had bilateral mastectomies. Rita, 56, was diagnosed seven years ago and was having what she describes as a 'mastectomy by degree' because of the number of lumps she had had removed. Jacqui, 50, had been diagnosed twice, once seven years ago and again five years ago. She had a single mastectomy.

Case study one: Nell

Nell, 58, is married and has two adult sons who no longer live at home. She lives in an outer suburb of Melbourne and is a retired medicolegal secretary. She and her husband migrated from England when they were first married and have been living in Melbourne ever since. Nell is proud of her experience of breast cancer and is very enthusiastic about being a part of my research. When I arrive at her house she has prepared many pages of notes retelling her experience in intricate detail. She even provides me with a list of the medication she has been on since her diagnosis. Initially she reads her story verbatim from her notes, delivering a literally scripted, factual list of events. Once I start interjecting a few questions she becomes distracted from her notes and tells me her story in a more natural way. Her husband pops in and out during the interview as did two workmen who were installing cable television. As we conduct the interview in the lounge room where the television is I ask a number of times if she would like to move to a quieter part of the house. Each time Nell refuses, telling me she is not embarrassed about her experience and feels quite comfortable. Although my request is motivated mostly by the fact that I am worried the dictaphone is not picking anything up because of the noise, we stay.

This insistence on staying while workmen tend to her television typifies the physical 'doing' of her post-surgical body during the interview. Nell's identity as a woman who has had breast cancer is something she is proud of and she emphasizes a liberated self. The interview also highlights the tensions of her new post-surgical self, as Nell is at once proud and public about her breast cancer yet finds it necessary to cover up her post-surgical body in order to fit a hegemonic feminine appearance.

Nell was diagnosed with breast cancer four years ago and had bilateral mastectomies followed by chemotherapy. She describes her diagnosis:

> I was on two-yearly mammograms, and afterwards I found out I should have been on yearly mammograms, because my mother had died of breast cancer in 1984. And she lived a lot longer than what she should have done with what she had. She was very brave. She was a widow and she coped all on her own. And when I went through what I went through I thought, how on earth did my mother ... and I cried for her, I didn't cry for me, I cried for her. And so I had my mammogram, two-yearly one, on a Saturday. And when I was on the table I said to the person who was doing the mammogram, can I have a look at it. And he sort of went, uhhh? Anyway I

made sure that I could have a look and as soon as I saw it I thought oh that doesn't look very spherical. And everyone went really quiet in the room. You know, there were three or four people there and nurses and technicians and all that sort of thing, and I just knew.

From the outset Nell's description and experience of her diagnosis is linked with her mother's. She articulates that her response to her own diagnosis was more of a response to her mother's experience, eliciting feelings of sympathy and bewilderment at her mother's coping all on her own. Nell wants to see for herself what her mammogram looks like. Her interpretation of it not looking very spherical and the quietness of the room lead her to draw her own conclusions, in her own words she says 'I just knew.'

So I got there about 2.00 pm and I was actually told about 6.00 pm. And when I went in there was this waiting room and it was just like a sausage factory, absolutely packed with all women, mostly middle aged and older women, and most were sitting there in fear. And there was me sitting there all gay and you know feeling perfectly calm and cool and collected, and I was feeling so sorry for all the other women who were absolutely frightened out of their minds. And then in the end I was the last one there at 6.00 pm and the surgeon sat me down and he put his head down, and I could just see he was so exhausted, and I knew what he was going to say. And he just said I am very sorry to tell you, you have cancer. And then he very quietly...he drew a diagram and he said he could do an incision in my right breast and that he could do me on Friday, which was three days away. So I said, fine. But then I told him I wanted a bilateral mastectomy. And I'd already told him that my mother had died of breast cancer and I didn't go into shock, you know, I stayed cool, calm and collected.

Nell situates herself as different from the other women in the waiting room – the 'sausage factory' – where women are lined up sitting in fear, waiting their turn to enter the doctor's office. Instead, she requests a bilateral mastectomy. In emphasizing how positively she reacts and distancing herself from the 'norm' she sets up the next part of her story. She makes sure I know where she is positioned within her narrative, as someone slightly superior, with a different story to tell. She emphasizes a level of self-importance, worthy of being listened to.

Nell goes on to contextualize her reaction in more detail:

And what had happened in about 1988, I was working at Monash Medical Centre and I went and saw the top breast surgeon there and when he was doing an examination he found one lump in my left breast and one lump in my right breast. And that night when I came home I said to Charlie [Husband], I have had such a shock today but I am all right now. I'm going to make a decision now about what I am going to do if I am told it is breast cancer, I want to make my mind up when I am not in shock. So I said to my husband, I want a bilateral mastectomy. I said life is too good. So when I went in and had the two lumps removed I said I didn't want to be woken up and told if I've got breast cancer and I wanted a bilateral mastectomy. But I woke up and they said oh no you are fine.

When Nell decides that she wants a bilateral mastectomy, the fact that the first lumps turn out to be benign does not deter her. There is a certain amount of disappointment in her construction of events. Nell is referred to genetic counselling, in which the risk of inheriting a genetic mutation and developing the disease are calculated and different types of risk management are discussed.

It came back that I was in a very low group. But they only took into account my family history and the fact that I only had my mother. They didn't take into account, because this is not part of the process, that I started my periods at ten, that I'd had no children of my own, both my sons were adopted, and then I had become pregnant but I contracted German measles at about four weeks so I had to have an abortion.

Nell is frustrated when her doctor concludes that 'family history' does not put her at a high enough risk to require a prophylactic mastectomy. A genetic predisposition forms part of what she sees as having caused her tumours. In addition Nell situates her cancer as linked to various reproductive choices and events that have occurred in her life: menstruating early, not having given birth to children of her own and having an abortion. She attempts to disentangle her lay beliefs about what causes cancer, no doubt drawn from popular health discourse on breast cancer, from medical expertise. Both of these are called upon to construct a meaningful account of the unfolding of events, integrating the cause and consequence of her illness into a new whole.[15] Nell attempts to take control of her body and fate by refusing to simply wait for her cancer to emerge. She positions herself as an agent of her illness and recovery, claiming responsibility for its causes and having a vital role in deciding on how to manage it.

> So when I was diagnosed it was not difficult because I'd already requested it. And he [the surgeon] obviously knew that I hadn't gone into shock or anything. He was in worse shock than I was. They hate giving the bad news... they find it really difficult, you know, he looked so drained and weary. Because it's like an epidemic now isn't it with the number of women who are getting it.

Nell presents herself as slightly superior to the battle weary doctor with whom she sympathizes. Her remark about the epidemic status of her disease distances her from her earlier claim of responsibility, instead situating herself, like other women with breast cancer, as a passive recipient of the disease.

Nell describes waking up from the mastectomy operation:

> I was just so well after I came around. And I think it was because I wasn't frightened, I wasn't scared, and I think in a way I was relieved. I think part of it was to... afterwards I went to my surgeon on one of my consultations, about the second or third time after the operation, and I said, I think some people might find my attitude a bit obscene, because I said I am really on a high, you know, I am really quite up beat and all this sort of thing. Oh he said, that's interesting, what we have found is that if you have had a history of breast cancer in the family it is like you have been standing on this landmine. So he said, when was your mother diagnosed and I said, in her 70s. He said, well you really have been standing on a landmine since then and he said when it goes off you are only too pleased to still be alive. And I think that's it.

Nell's surgeon articulates for her that her cancer is a 'landmine' that has exploded. After a nearly 30-year family history of breast cancer, she is now no longer at risk. This validation of her feelings elicits more emphasis on her positivity towards the operation. After a long period of constant surveillance of her body, the cancer has finally 'gone off' and she can now move on with her life with relative safety.

> I lifted the sheets up and I had a look but I mean it was just flat. But it didn't sort of horrify me or anything. And I have never felt disfigured.

And that was another thing before I actually had the operation. Charlie was not really in favour of me having a bilateral mastectomy, he felt that I should only have the section taken out. And Charlie actually did a lovely thing to me the night before I had the operation, before I went into hospital. He said to me, I have changed my mind on bilateral mastectomy. And he said, oh yes, I think if you have both of them removed you haven't got one left to remind you of what the other one looked like. Now wasn't that lovely of him to think of, you know, I hadn't thought of that. And also I hadn't thought about that it's much easier to fit two prostheses than make the one look the same as the other.

Nell has 'never felt disfigured', implying that perhaps she could. Her husband's suggestion that she will not have one breast to remind her of the other reassures Nell and brings her attention to the fact it will now be easier to get two prostheses to 'fit' instead of trying to match one to a natural breast. Even before the operation her post-surgical body is framed as temporary, having to be returned to its prior state, if only in appearance to others. Nell talks about her mastectomy with reference to how she *does not* feel – she is *not* horrified and does *not* feel disfigured. There are only negative associations to talk about her corporeal self, highlighting a lack of positive discourse available to talk about the post-surgical body.

In keeping with her positioning as in control of her illness and recovery, Nell expresses concern about her recommended follow up treatment:

I didn't understand how others who looked like me and were similar in age were getting chemotherapy. So I had this huge argument with my surgeon regarding it, and he said to me chemotherapy wouldn't help me. And I didn't understand why but it was because my cancer was hormone negative and I thought that was because I was no longer having periods. So I didn't understand. I mean I am not stupid but because you are not in the ... and I mean I thought I was quite clued up because I had worked in the medical [field] so I asked the right questions. But it's not a state of where your body is at it's a state of the actual cancer itself.

Nell is concerned about her follow-up treatment, or lack of it, because she sees others who are of similar age and 'look like me' who are having chemotherapy, whereas she is not. She is defensive about misunderstanding the discrepancy between her body and 'the cancer itself'. This has implications for Nell as she struggles to retain control over what is happening to her.

> So I went and saw Tara [oncologist] and she sat down with me and she sort of laid out the statistics for me and I would only gain perhaps five per cent benefit from having chemo instead of the . . . if my cancer had been hormone positive, and people in my age group weren't really being given chemo but they were just starting to give people in my age group chemo. And so she then said to me that I could have a six month or a three month [course]. And she was lovely. At the end of the consultation, because I never really said did you think it was worth it or anything like that, I think she knew I was just a black and white person. Because I said to her, I said I want the AC chemo, the one where you lose your hair and everything, because I have got a feeling that if you have the hardest chemo that there is then it will kill off more cancer cells. And she turned around to me and she said, that is not so, but she said, I have a gut feeling like you do. She was lovely.

In separating her body from the cancer she produces a theory that if she has the 'hardest chemo' it will 'kill off more cells'. Although it is diffi-cult to ascertain whether Tara the oncologist simply complies with Nell's request because she understands she is a 'black and white person' or if there is actually more to it, the end result means Nell holds Tara in high regard, emphasizing how 'lovely' she is. From Nell's account Tara shares Nell's 'gut feeling' that chemotherapy is the way to go.

> I mean I didn't have radiotherapy because I didn't have a part, you only have radiation therapy when you have a part taken away. But the huge advantage of me having chemotherapy means that I now have two different specialists looking after me so it's not just the one. And they both have different ideas and pick up different things. But I am not saying that they would pick up that I have got secondaries. I think I'd be the first person to know. But it's lovely having two different personalities because there is one thing you can discuss with one and there are different things you can discuss with the other.

Nell reiterates this faith in her knowledge of her body and the advan-tages of having chemotherapy.

And I was feeling so well after I had my chemo. Now a friend of mine has just had the same chemo and she has to be hospitalized one full day after and she is in bed for one whole week. And I was just nothing like that. Now after I had my first dose I went back to my oncologist and I said because I am so well can I have an increased dose.

Nell interprets her feeling 'so well' after the treatment as her body telling her she needs 'more chemo'. Her understanding of the treatment is that the sicker it makes you, the better job it must be doing; thus she interprets feeling well as meaning not enough cells are being killed. Relying on her body to tell her means she can assume responsibility and control. Nell describes her body and self as working together, she listens to what her body is telling her and in return her body responds positively by becoming well. Nell simultaneously draws on biomedical and social understandings of sickness and health.

I asked my surgeon what my life expectancy was and he would not answer. He got quite angry because he said, you can't say. But I am a person who likes to know so I phoned CanHelp and I got the information i.e. that I had a 45 per cent chance of living four-and-a-half years because of where my cancer got to. I would have been really pissed off if I had died before four-and-a-half years but I am going to make it because I have lived four years and three months.

Nell really has her sights set on this timeline, exclaiming how annoyed she would be if she did not make it, now that she is only two months from the survivor status that timeline has granted her.

I have been so lucky because I have never felt disfigured and I still run around the house naked. The only time I do find it difficult is I absolutely love swimming and I like sun dresses so I have to wear a bra where it doesn't show and the dress so it doesn't show and the bathers so it doesn't show, and it's quite difficult. When you bend down and you have got bathers on it can often sort of hang down so they can see that you haven't got any boobs. And I am not worried for myself, I mean I couldn't care less but other people like children or elderly people can get highly embarrassed . . . my son has made me some prostheses out of shoulder pads and he has sewn them into my bathing costume and they are really quite safe.

In commenting that she has 'never felt disfigured' Nell positions herself as different to how she assumes she should feel. She states that she does not worry about her body image for herself, but for others, as 'they' can get 'highly embarrassed'. The shoulder pads that her son has sewn into her bathing costume are 'safe' not only because they will not fall out, but because no one can tell she has no breasts. Nell is herself 'safe' from the stare of others and the embarrassment she feels she may cause.

> I like to look...you know the funny thing is I never spend money on hair or my face or my skin, but I like nice clothes. And I still feel sexy. So I suppose it's part of my image...I mean I was just so thankful that I wasn't in my 20s or 30s or 40s because I have always been quite slim and not bad looking. I know it sounds terrible but we are all vain aren't we? And I never had big boobs. So there isn't any problem. But I never worry what other people think...Now another friend of mine, she has just had a bilateral mastectomy, and she said that her aim is to walk out without anything, without prostheses! But I'd never ever thought of it. I'd never thought of going without. And I still don't think that I would. This is really the first time I have thought about it. And I suppose I should make the statement, I am saying it would be nice but that's not me, I like to look sexy and nice. Although I am 58 coming up 59 I probably no longer look sexy. And also I know it upsets people.

Wearing a prosthesis equates to looking 'sexy and nice'. It has never occurred to her to go 'without', although she feels this is a statement she should perhaps be making. Nell wears the prostheses so as not to upset people; however, she also says she does not worry what other people think. Although she tells me she 'still runs around the house naked' she wears her prosthesis and bra to bed.

> And that's for Charlie to cuddle me because it just feels more natural. When he cuddles my body and it's just my bare ribs it just doesn't feel normal whereas when he cuddles me like that, you know, it just feels normal.

Nell's narrative is made up of constant distinctions between how she thinks she should feel and how she actually feels. In repeatedly comparing herself to others, she is empowered by exceeding expectations of the norm, feeling 'so well' after the mastectomy and chemotherapy. She positions herself outside of the norm, as not being part of the 'sausage factory'. But Nell also wants to be part of this collective – in getting chemo like the others of her age.

Both fate and self-determinacy play a role in Nell's cancer. She situates it as both a foreign entity that is independent of her body yet she also locates cancer inherently within her body and as part of who she is – a woman with a genetic history of breast cancer.

Her illness occurs in a context of family history of breast cancer, where cancer means death. In recent years attention has been paid to the ways women experience the ambiguities and uncertainties of being 'at risk' for breast cancer.[16] Kavanagh and Broom (1998) have identified three categories of risk: environmental risks which are due to something that *happens* to a person; lifestyle risks which occur because of something a person does or does not *do*; and embodied risks that say something about who the person *is*. Embodied or corporeal risks pose a 'threat from within' (1998: 442) and as such women have limited possibilities for dealing with the hazard. Kavanagh and Broom suggest that because corporeal risk involves threat from one's own body there is a resulting dissociation between body and self: 'Her body could be dissected, hazardous parts identified and removed, while the self remained – no longer under threat from the body' (1998: 442).

Hallowell (2000: 155) argues that the adoption of an 'at-risk' identity has profound implications for the way women conceive of the self and their bodies. The metaphor of the landmine correlates to Hallowell's research which conceives the 'at risk' genetic body as a 'dangerous body'. Within this discourse cancer is constructed as a silent and deadly disease, just like a landmine, sitting there waiting for something to trigger it off. It is 'the danger within, a malign agent'.[17] The military metaphors Nell uses to describe her cancer and treatment, both the cancer as a 'landmine' and the chemo that 'kills off' cells, refer to broader cultural narratives of the body and immune system.[18] Hallowell identifies prophylactic mastectomy as enabling women to regain control of their body by disposing of the dangerous parts – the breasts. But Nell does not just link it to her family history, she is frustrated when the doctors do not see it as linked to her other reproductive health choices.

Nell produces a knowledge of her body that lies outside of biomedicine, stating she will know before the specialists do if she has secondaries. This knowledge is coupled with popular health ideas about causes, namely reproductive health problems. Discussions are thus 'packaged in a rhetoric of culpability that produces a particular kind of gendered guilt: one contracts breast cancer because one has not made the "proper" . . .

reproductive choices'.[19] Yadlon (1997) argues that breast cancer discourse implies that the way to prevent the disease is to follow dominant codes of femininity.

Twice Nell emphasizes having never felt disfigured taking pride in the fact she still runs around the house naked. However, she wears prostheses so as to not embarrass others and wears a bra and prostheses to bed to feel more natural and normal for her husband. This contradiction between not feeling disfigured yet covering up symbolizes a disconnection between body and self. What she *feels* is different from what she *does*.

Nell's account is embedded in broader cultural narratives of the body and sickness, discourses of risk and genetics, and she draws on these readily available scripts to articulate her experience. She uses these narratives to both set herself apart from the norm and situate herself firmly within it. The themes of normality, fate and self-determinacy all have implications for her sense of self and the performance of her post-surgical body. The liberation she feels when the breast cancer has 'exploded' is superseded by her need to maintain a watchful eye over her body, for the sake of others, in making sure no one sees that she has no breasts. Feeling 'safe' and 'natural' and 'normal' are enabled by the use of prostheses. She is at once proud and unashamed of her breastless body as it symbolizes a new self free of cancer and cancer-risk, and at the same time she is constrained from showing off this new body publicly as it risks embarrassing others.

Throughout her account Nell situates herself as a slightly superior self, as being healthier and tougher and on the whole dealing with breast cancer better than other women. I am thus slightly surprised that Nell does not make a decision not to wear a prosthesis and not be a part of the norm. Nell acknowledges this contradiction; however, she sees it as too big a sacrifice, to not look and feel 'sexy and nice'. As liberated as she emphasizes herself to be, she is unable to align the body she performs in public and in her own bedroom with the body she talks of so proudly. She is constrained by the expectation and risk of upsetting others and not feeling natural to her husband and as such cannot feel normal without the aid of prostheses.

Case study two: Rita

Rita, 56, is divorced with two adult daughters. She was a social worker until her many health problems meant she had to resign. Rita was diagnosed with breast cancer seven years ago. She had a lumpectomy, chemotherapy and radiotherapy and since her initial diagnosis has had four more lumps removed, all of which have been benign. Her last lumpectomy was three months ago. She spoke to me in her home in Melbourne.

While many of the interviews I conducted were more like conversations between myself and the participant, I did little except nod during my morning with Rita. Our meeting began with my asking her to tell me about when she found out she had breast cancer and what followed was two and a half hours of uninterrupted monologue. This is part of her story:

> I found out by accident. I was going to my doctor because I've got chronic fatigue syndrome, which started with a bout of glandular fever 13 years ago. I was going to my GP, and talking to him about that. I guess I was starting to go through menopause and starting to have hot flushes, and lots of things like that, because it was really uncomfortable. So I went to him and asked him about HRT, and he said, oh yeah, we can just put you straight on it and you won't have to go through menopause, and everything will be fine, etc etc. I worked at the arthritis foundation, and they recommended HRT for women to prevent osteoporosis, but reading up about it there was also stuff about, it can make cancer worse. And I already had a thyroid problem, so I asked to go to an Endocrinologist before I went on to the HRT, just to see if that was OK, and what difference it would make to my thyroid condition etc etc.

From the outset Rita's experience of breast cancer is linked to her many other health problems: chronic fatigue syndrome, glandular fever, symptoms of menopause and problems with her thyroid. Unhappy with her regular GP she seeks another opinion, this time from a woman:

> She [the GP] examined my breasts really thoroughly, which had not happened ever. She found a thickening that I hadn't recognized as a lump, because I've always had ropey breasts. I'd been to the doctors a few times thinking I had a lump, and they'd say oh no, you've just got ropey breasts. So she picked this up, and she said 'is that normal?' And I said I really don't know, um, but I sort of knew it was there, but didn't know it was anything different. So she sent me off for a mammogram the next day. So I went and had the mammogram, and they gave me the films to take back to my doctor. I ripped them open in the car park [laugh], so I was sitting in the car park, and it said something along the lines of 'something or other, something or other, a thickening, very likely to be malignant because of such and

such'. So I knew it was likely to be that, so I went to my [regular] GP the next day, and he had a look at it and said 'oh, it doesn't look like much to me'. [pause]. But I already knew the truth. I'd read the report.

Rita's 'ropey breasts' have caused her false alarms before, confusing her about what is 'normal' for her breasts. Her GP dismisses the mammogram report; however, Rita already knows the 'truth'. She positions herself in her narrative as being victimized by a series of health problems and then by a dismissive doctor. Rita then goes to see the surgeon:

And he was the loveliest, kindest, sweetest man, and he sort of took a look at the films, and examined me, and said 'well I don't really know what it is but we'll have to have a look, take it out' . . . So I went in and I was so terrified, and I thought I was handling this very well, but when they examined me they sent me off to have a cardiograph because my heart was beating so fast they thought something might be wrong [laugh].

The surgeon who takes her concerns seriously elicits a very positive appraisal from Rita, highlighting that this is not normally how she feels she is treated. Her fear and anxiety about what is happening is medicalized as she is sent off to have a cardiograph because of her racing heart.

I came round after the surgery, and he was there at the end of the bed, and he said you know, it is malignant. And I just burst into tears, and I said to my daughter, 'I love you so much, I don't want to leave you' and she said 'I know'. And we both had a big cry. So that was the finding out part, yeah . . . I can't remember what I knew. I was very innocent about the whole thing at that stage.

Rita's recollection of the 'finding out part' leads her to reflect that she was 'very innocent' about it all at that point. This innocence reflects a time of uncertainty and naivety about the process she had to go through and feelings of vulnerability and anxiety towards the medical profession.

My auntie by marriage to my mother had had a radical mastectomy years and years ago. I knew that she suffered really, really acute pain after it, and I'd heard a really interesting show years and years ago, which said that a lumpectomy plus radiotherapy was as good as a mastectomy, you didn't have to have a mastectomy. So I went in knowing that, not wanting to have a mastectomy because I thought it would be more painful, and I chose really to have the lump [removed]. He came in and said what he would do, what he called a quadrantectomy, so the tumour was in the upper, outer quadrant of the right breast, which is the worst place because it's closest to your lymph nodes. So he explained that he would remove that quadrant of the breast and the lymph nodes.

The production of breast cancer knowledge based on popular health discourse on cancer and its treatment has great significance for Rita. She bases her decision on her knowledge of her auntie's acute pain from her radical mastectomy some years earlier, and a television program which outlines an apparent ideal treatment. It is her fear of pain that largely motivates this decision, an attempt to avoid further suffering in the context of her other ailments.

So I went back into hospital and I had what I just said done, and I was absolutely amazed at how incredibly painful it was. It was terribly, terribly, terribly painful. Not so much in the breast, but where they had removed the lymph nodes under my arm. It felt as if, as if they had pulled out half of my arm. Unfortunately when I had the surgery, that particular surgery, it was just before Easter, I kept asking could I see a social worker, because I was just feeling so traumatized, and I've done social work myself, I just wanted to talk to someone about all of the issues. Not just the feeling terrified issues, but financial issues. What do you do when you can't work? All that sort of thing. Nobody came. The physiotherapist was supposed to come and see me everyday. He came once and said you've got to get exercising, and left. I didn't see him again. Then in the end I was sent home really with nothing.

An intelligent, informed woman, Rita has insight into the issues that are raised with surgery and breast cancer. She feels abandoned by the medical profession as she goes home with no support, with 'nothing'. She positions herself as a victim of bad timing and intense pain.

Later she revisits the hospital to collect pathology results and is again filled with uncertainty.

It was a small tumour – it was only one centimetre – there was nothing in my lymph nodes, they were all clear. So it was only, he didn't actually explain much about it, only that it was really small. So I didn't have a clue what should happen after that. The first thing he tried to do was enroll me in a trial of a new drug, which was to stop your ovaries from working, which would then cut down on the oestrogen supply to your breast, and if the tumour was there and it didn't have oestrogen it probably wouldn't grow. But it seemed to me that was ridiculous because I was menopausal anyway, I couldn't really see why I would be in a trial that would cause menopause if that's what was happening to me anyway. And I refused that [participation in the trial], and he got really offended and angry about.

Rita's refusal to be enrolled in the clinical trial causes resentment from her doctor. To her the doctor is not listening to her, not taking into consideration her understanding of what is going on with her body. As she attempts to assert some control over what is happening she is left confused and upset. Her resistance to the medical trial further positions her at odds with the medical professionals she has to deal with. A power struggle emerges between Rita and her doctor over who knows her body the most, and who knows what is best for it.

He [the surgeon] said oh yes, but you're only in the middle of menopause you're not right through it yet. But it didn't seem right to me, and I knew I had, from the first time I met him, just a core distrust about him. I really didn't like him. I suppose by the way he treated my fears in a really non compassionate way, as if I was stupid for feeling frightened. So then I said, what else? He said, well, some people say that I come in too strongly, but I would say you should have chemotherapy, and some people would say that's overreacting, but that's what I think you should get. So not knowing anything, I said alright. So this was a Friday and I booked in for about 10.30am on the Monday. But I still didn't trust him, I really didn't trust him at all. So I went in on the Monday and had my first dose of chemotherapy.

Rita's fears and uncertainty are overpowered by the surgeon. Although she has strong negative feelings about him her assumed lack of knowledge makes her feel she has no grounds to argue. Even though her senses alert her to potential problems she is once again relegated to the mercy of 'experts'. As her narrative unfolds she reveals the consequences of going against her gut feelings.

I found the experience of the chemotherapy absolutely terrifying. I'm still not sure whether it was just me, but they couldn't find a vein first of all. They said I had really bad veins and that took ages to actually get it in. But then during the chemotherapy [I had] the most weird sensation, and I found out since that it is normal, but I didn't know then, is that it actually causes a burning sensation as it goes around your body and when it hits your genitals it was a really, really, really hot and burning feeling. And I also knew because of the chronic fatigue syndrome that I've got that I'm hyper-allergic to things. So I was lying there worrying myself sick about this terrible feeling thinking something's gone wrong, I'm going to die. And then I came home, and I actually felt high as a kite. I couldn't sleep. I found out later, that's because they put cortisone in it, but I didn't know then. And I thought what's happening to me, am I going crazy? Is this normal? Feeling really shocking about the whole thing.

Her uncertainty about whether her reaction to the treatment is 'just me' alienates Rita. Her 'bad veins', the 'burning' of the chemotherapy, her concern about being 'hyper-allergic' and then subsequently feeling 'high as a kite' lead her to question whether she is 'crazy' or 'normal'. Rita is situated amongst all of this distress, unable to manage what is happening to her.

I was so distressed by the whole thing that I thought I've got to try and find a way out of this. So I rang the anti-cancer council and spoke to some nurses there, who were very surprised that I wasn't having radiotherapy. Then I went along to a [...] cancer support group meeting. I borrowed a book from them, which mentioned all the side effects of different cancer treatments, including chemo-therapy. Including damage to your veins, liver damage, damage to lots of your body's organs, and it said unless you have no other choice, don't have chemotherapy. So it seemed to me that with a small lump and nothing in the lymph nodes, perhaps that was too much treatment, more than I needed. So, just because I'm a social worker and I know how to do it, and I've done it before, I actually rang up the State Library of Victoria and got them to do a literature search for me. So I did that, so I had all the journal materials and I read it, and it was really clear that in my situation what you should be having is radiotherapy, just to get rid of any local malignant cells, you should be seeing if the lump was hormone receptor positive, and if it was you should be having tamoxifen for two years, and even if it wasn't hormone receptor positive, you should still have tamoxifen anyway. That there was an 80 per cent chance that I would never have a recurrence, because it was small and not in the lymph nodes.

Giving me any other sort of treatment would add about three per cent to an 80 per cent chance. And not having radiotherapy was also a big risk factor for having a recurrence.

Using her skills and knowledge of resources as a social worker Rita begins to regain some control. This production of knowledge enables a shift from being a vulnerable patient to a capable and empowered woman.

So I went along to my GP and I said look, would you read this for me and see if I am interpreting this correctly? I mean I was sure I was, but you know. I came back the next day and he said to me, you're so lucky that you read this, I've been onto another oncologist that I send people to, and he's absolutely furious too, because you're getting totally the wrong treatment. And you must have radio-therapy, and the chemotherapy is just not warranted. And he said that oncologist is in big trouble. So I then went along to a new oncologist who was very reassuring, who said there's an 80 per cent chance that the surgery itself would have cured it, but he said you never know whether you're in the 20 people out of a hundred or you're the 80 people out of a hundred. Statistics are OK, but you never know which bit you're going to be in. So he said well, I've booked you in for radiotherapy, and he said we'll put you on tamoxifen anyway.

Rita questions her own judgment and seeks 'expert' opinion to double check her interpretation of the literature. Her findings point to the fact that her initial distrust of the doctor in recommending the chemo-therapy were grounded in reality – she was being given the wrong treat-ment. In doing this she is able to take back some of what had been taken from her:

So that was in a way a real turning point for me, because I really felt as though I was at the mercy of all of these people, and not under-standing what was going on. But from that stage I felt as though I was back in control of my own life, and my own body again. And that I could read this material, and I could understand it, and I did read it, and I did understand it, and I was right, and I was able to say I don't want this oncologist I'll have this one. And that really was just a turning point, taking charge of my own life again. And feeling that well, whatever happens to me, I can read about it, and I can understand it, and people will listen to me, and realize that I can.

This 'turning point' signifies a shift to empowerment; a transition from passive recipient of the treatment and medical expertise to becoming an agent of her illness and recovery. Knowledge enables her to reclaim her self and body, allowing her to put her experience in perspective and give it coherence. She can determine with self-confidence what she will or will not do. Rita's research vindicates her instincts about the surgeon and the treatment giving her faith in herself. She positions herself as both intelligent and capable.

> But what's happened after the radiotherapy, and I didn't know that this would happen at the time, is that scar tissue forms in your breast, and that scar tissue forms lumps, so you really don't know if you've got a new lump or not, or is it just scar tissue from the radiotherapy. It also causes the most peculiar sensation on the skin. If you touch the area where you had the radiotherapy it's almost numb, but not quite, and it's the most unpleasant experience, touching the bare skin where you've had the radiotherapy. It doesn't matter to me, because I'm not in a sexual relationship with anyone, it's just something I find unpleasant, even when you're washing yourself. But for a lot of my friends who are married, the fact that they can't feel their breasts being touched has caused huge problems for them.

The radiotherapy has far-reaching implications for Rita, both physically and emotionally. She dismisses the 'unpleasant' sensation of her skin as unimportant in the absence of a sexual relationship. She is alienated from her breasts, unable to touch them. Of greater importance to Rita and her story are the lumps which have developed from the scar tissue:

> I've had three lumps removed from my breast since then. The same breast. Each time I went along to get them to have a look at the lump, and they'd say we don't know what it is until we take it out, so I'd go along and have it taken out. And each time it's turned out to be fatty necrosis . . . the tissue that's been killed by the radiotherapy. And it just dies, and then it just sits in your breast, and in some people it causes lumps, in others it's just dead cells, but in me it caused lumps. So each time I've got one of these I've gone along, not knowing whether it was a recurrence, and not knowing whether it was OK. The last one was only three months ago, I went along to the surgeon and he said, this is so different to what you've had before, we better take it seriously, we need to do it quickly.

So I went in and had it done, feeling absolutely terrified. And I really coped alright. I organized things at home, did everything. And people said, oh gee you're really fantastic, because I went into hospital and I got the results which were that it was really OK, it was more fatty necrosis. And I went into the deepest trough of depression. It was like, I was keeping going while the adrenalin was running when I didn't know, and when I knew I really felt quite, [pauses, begins to cry, pauses] it amazed me that I felt quite suicidal. There was one part of me that was saying this is going to be happening for the rest of your life, you're going to get more lumps and you're going to keep going back, and you're never going to know. The surgeon had said to me, you're just one of those people this happens to. For the rest of my life I'm going to be going back having lumps removed and not knowing what they are. And it was really quite terrifying, because part of me wanted to give up, and part of me didn't. And it sounds quite psychotic I know.

The scar tissue that 'just dies' and then 'just sits' in her breast is a major locus of fear and anxiety. Although a time of uncertainty, Rita positions herself as in control, able to manage her household and work and generally keeps things together. There is a sense of routine to the tests that have now happened a number of times. She is able to play an active role preparing for a potential positive diagnosis of breast cancer. However, instead of her negative result eliciting a happy response she is deeply depressed by yet another false alarm. The surgeon depersonalizes her experience by slotting her into a collective of 'people this happens to', refusing her any space to feel sorry for herself and grieve. Because the 'result was fine' Rita is not allowed legitimate status as 'sick' and thus feels she cannot explain to people why she feels depressed and suicidal.

I've talked to other women who have had radiotherapy who have also said they've had side effects. The aching in their bones and their face, some people have had heart problems. Nobody told me about that. Nobody told me that that was a risk. Surgeons have been really nice to me, and the radical mastectomy would be terrible, I've read about that and you wouldn't want that. They try to do the right things by us now by conserving our breasts, but in a way they are also caught up in the social ideology of what breasts are for, and if I'd known all of the side effects I would have chosen a mastectomy. But they all tried so hard to keep a good cosmetic effect, when that wasn't an issue for me. I just wanted to stay alive. I would rather just have the mastectomy. And I get lymphoedema in my arms, and that causes me pain. So I'm often in quite a lot of pain in my arms and near my breast, from the lymph glands being removed. I think there needs to be some rethinking about what you present to women, because nobody ever presented a mastectomy to me as a choice, nobody ever told me the truth about the side effects of radiotherapy. But I think we have to rethink the choices that women are being given, that it's not everyone's choice to conserve their breasts at all costs, and it wasn't for me it was just I thought if I had the lumpectomy I'd have less pain [laugh]. But I didn't know.

Withholding the 'truth' about the effects of treatment joins a long list of things that Rita feels were kept from her. This 'truth' includes aching in the bones and face, possible heart problems and pain caused by lymphoedema. She sees this as a trade-off for the 'good cosmetic effect' that she never actually requested. She believes that the surgeons try to do the 'right thing' by women, by conserving breasts. The 'social ideology' that the surgeons are 'caught up in' that Rita alludes to focuses on 'what breasts are for', presumably as symbols of sexuality, femininity and identity. She situates herself as naïve in not requesting the mastectomy. She is angry that it was not given to her as a choice yet situates herself as ultimately responsible. Earlier in her narrative Rita articulates that she chose the lumpectomy to avoid pain; however, now she says she was not given a choice. Instead she feels duped by a patriarchal medical system. This contradiction highlights the constant power struggle consistent in her account. The fluctuating positioning of the self in her own narrative further illustrates this point.

Rita then goes on to tell me the sad story of her life before her cancer diagnosis. In doing this she contextualizes her illness experience, associating breast cancer with these things:

I have a really terrible background. I suffered sexual abuse and physical abuse as a child, and that I think, I've done a lot of looking at people who get chronic fatigue syndrome, and I definitely had glandular fever, but why did it not go away? One of the reasons seems to be that people who've been through that sort of situation, I mean I married an alcoholic who was verbally abusive, I had a daughter who, the stress was enormous because the condition was so rare, I mean she actually sued some doctors who operated on her without an anesthetic. It's been one stress in my life after another and in my reading, it suggests that your immune system just gets depleted, your adrenals just get exhausted, so you're prone to get things that you might not get if you hadn't have had all those things in your past. I think that's all involved with that and I think I got the cancer two years after these horrible men operated on my daughter without anesthetic, and it was such an horrific time I can't describe to you how terrible it was. My feelings, my dealing with the cancer all gets involved with all of these other things that are going on.

Her medical history – the chronic fatigue syndrome and glandular fever – is connected to her personal life history – sexual, physical and verbal abuse, an alcoholic husband, her daughter's major health problems – she describes them 'one stress after another' as culminating in the depletion of her immune system and exhaustion of adrenals. To Rita this is the cause of her cancer and directly implicates her interpretation of the illness experience. Her reading of medical and popular health is produced and organized within and against this frame.

It's really only in the last two weeks, that I've realized that this is grief. And why do I feel like I want to cry all the time? Because I'm grieving for a state of, I was never innocent, but a state of innocence that I had before I had cancer, and that I will never be able to get back. See there's been no cancer in my family, I was shocked that I got it, but in another way I wasn't surprised because of all the, I mean I know, I've worked in child protective services, and I actually know that abuse and all of those things affect you in later life, and I know all of that stuff. So I wasn't surprised to get a few of these illnesses, you know what I mean? But, it's like you lose that sense of innocence that everything will be alright, I mean you're constantly frightened the whole time, that you know, you get a pain in your knee and you think Oh God, it's cancer in my bones.

Rita articulates a lost state of innocence that she can never regain because of her cancer. This innocence that she is grieving for symbolizes a sense that 'everything will be alright', that she can become well again. What has been taken from her, and what she is grieving for, is the fact that she will never be 'well again' but will be forever existing in the space between 'well' and 'sick'. In this space she is denied the privileges of being either healthy and 'normal' or legitimately ill, getting sympathy from others and relief from her responsibilities.

So the cancer is there in your mind every time you feel something, and it's like, is this a recurrence? Does this mean I have secondaries? I'm going to be going back to the doctor having lumps removed for the rest of my life, I'm sort of having a mastectomy by degree. I really, just as I'm talking to you I'm thinking, that the next time it happens you know do I just say to them, just do a mastectomy and get it over and done with. I really don't want to be going through this again and again. I said to him [the doctor] once I might as well have a mastectomy, and he said 'Oh no'. It's like, they are all being really kind to us but, in a way it's not a kindness to assume that they know what you want. It's not a kindness at all. And in these men, they are mostly all men, being really kind conserving our breasts for us, they're all assuming that they know what we want, but they are assuming that they know what any individual wants. So they might be right about women as a group, but they are not necessarily right about each of us as an individual.

Hyden (1997: 156) suggests:

Through the narrative, the experience of illness is *articulated*, especially the suffering associated with illness. By arranging the illness symptoms and events in temporal order and relating them to other events in our lives, a unified context is constructed and coherence is established. (original emphasis)

More than simply a contextualization of her illness experience, Rita situates breast cancer as almost a logical conclusion to all that has happened to her prior to diagnosis. Rita's account is located within a long history of health problems and her diagnosis does not surprise her. She makes a connection between the relentless stress in her life and her depleted immune system, stating that her body is 'exhausted' and she is therefore 'prone' to get things. To her, cancer is directly linked to her abusive background. Rita has a history of being violated and betrayed by men, by an abusive parent and husband and by the medical profession. In both instances a potentially 'safe' environment turns out to be a locus of pain and fear. Rita's account is a narrative of her body's response to years of abuse and stress. She positions herself as unable to control what happens to her and at the same time as ultimately responsible.

The narrative enables her to be reflexive about the 'turning point' where she takes charge of treatment decision making, but she is overwhelmed by her grief and suffering. Her narrative is driven by tensions between feelings of abandonment, pain, fate and control.

The reframing of her identity as neither 'sick' nor 'well' creates a constant strain as she is unable to reconcile her body and self amongst the grief, pain and struggle. Rita is alienated by her lack of access to legitimate status as 'sick' as she has repeated recurrences of lumps that turn out to be benign. Being caught between 'sick' and 'not sick' creates a tension that has serious implications for her sense of self and emotional stability. She contemplates suicide because of the stress this causes, illustrating the impact this has on her.

Case study three: Jacqui

Jacqui, 50, lives in Queanbeyan, just outside of Canberra. She has never married or had children and although she started her career as a nurse she is now a public servant. Jacqui was first diagnosed with breast cancer seven years before resulting in a single mastectomy and radio-therapy. She had a recurrence two years later but has had many lumps removed over the past nine years.

> My first diagnosis was on my 43rd birthday. I had a tumour in my left breast. I had a biopsy and that came out malignant. So I had to toss up between a mastectomy or a lumpectomy – even though I don't know what a breast lump feels like – or nothing. And I am not good at doing nothing. So that wasn't an option. And I didn't want to lose a breast. So it was a lumpectomy. And the tumour was very, very small, it was only about 2cm, so it was only just starting to shoot its legs and grow. I had a wide incision, they went in and took more tissue out and removed all my lymph glands on the left side. They were clear. But I had follow up, they followed up with radio-therapy. So that was okay. I thought right, been there done that, let's get on with it. The next year I had I think tumours in both breasts.

Early in her narrative Jacqui positions herself as having an active role in treatment decision making. Her 'let's get on with it' attitude after the surgery and treatment is halted by a second diagnosis the following year.

> Initially I got mastitis and I wanted to know why, because I haven't had children, I hadn't lactated. There was no reason for a bacteria to get in or whatever it was. And I wouldn't accept it when the doctors, three doctors said, oh these things happen. I said, no, my body's

telling me something. He said, okay go and have a mammogram. And that's how I found out. So I've asked different surgeons about it, and they said, oh mastitis doesn't cause cancer. And I'm saying, no, I'm not saying it causes it, I am saying the mastitis or the infection grew around a tumour and that alerted me to there was something wrong. So that's why I haven't felt any lumps. Because my breasts were never lumpy. They used to swell up before periods and get very sore, but they were never lumpy.

Jacqui links her illness to health problems that occurred prior to her diagnosis. She refuses to accept the doctors' dismissal of the cause of her cancer and instead offers her interpretation. She attempts to situate these events in a unified context. In locating the birthplace of her tumour she is able to construct coherence and order the chaos of what is happening to her.

I had the lumpectomy, radiotherapy as well. And once the burning from the radiotherapy had healed I went back to yoga and I started swimming and did everything as normal. There was a lot of emotional stuff to cope with. I had to get on with things. And then the next year I had one in each breast. And they did biopsies on those and they were both benign. So that was rightio, let's get going again. And then the next year I had a malignant one in my right breast, so they took that out. No need for another...I mean they were getting smaller and smaller because I was checked up so often. And then the next year I went for my checkup a bit early and I had another one in my right breast. So I moved down here and then I went back to Sydney and they did an ultrasound on my right breast and I was riddled with tiny tumours.

Again Jacqui emphasizes her need to 'get on with things' and 'get going again'. In doing so she positions herself as in control, as experiencing a temporary setback that she is capable of over coming.

I've never had big breasts but they were just...they were a part of me. You know you lose a finger...it's a part of you, it's going to affect your life. I think to me breasts are a symbol of nurturing. They are certainly a symbol of your sexuality. And I liked them. They were small, but I never thought that I'd like bigger breasts. They were quite comfortable. I could not wear a bra quite comfortably. And sleep on my stomach quite comfortably. And then of course once they were threatened I liked them even more. But when it came to having [the mastectomy]…my left breast is the one that has got holes in it, whereas most of the scar tissue around the right breast is on the bottom. But I didn't want to lose it. And I'd obviously been fighting not to lose it. Just remove the tumours, see how it goes. And then they rang me, they wanted me to come back and have more mammograms on my left breast because they thought I had another tumour there. And that wiped me out. I said no not that. But that was okay. And when I saw the ultrasound on my right breast I said you can say what you like but I can see that. I said I have got a really small breast but there must be 100 of those things in there. So I said it's going to have to come off.

For Jacqui, her breasts are a part of who she is, more than simply a part of her physical body; they are symbols of nurturing (although she has not had any children) and sexuality. These common associations locate the importance of breasts to identity and a sense of self. Jacqui fought to save her right breast, but had a mastectomy and although her left breast has 'holes' in it, she does not want to lose it. She describes herself as in control of the decision to have the mastectomy independent of the doctor's opinion. She is eager to emphasize the active role she has in the decision-making process.

When I had my mastectomy a social worker came to see me and I had a lot of other problems as well. There was a lot going on apart from just the physical. A friend died of cancer the day I had surgery. A lot of issues with my mother who came up to look after me. And all of that. I have got a very complex relationship with my mother. So you know, there were a lot of other things going on. So I was battling and coping. Getting on with it. Getting better. Getting out of hospital.

Jacqui's illness experience is situated amongst other events in her life, breast cancer just another thing she must battle and overcome.
  She describes looking at her mastectomy for the first time:

I was actually very proud of myself and just really consciously looked at it. Up until then I'd sort of get out of the shower and turn my back to the mirror and duck out again. And then one day just sort of turned around and had a good look. I thought, oh well, that's it it's not so bad after all. And there have been other times now when I have, you know. There are times when I think it would be really nice just to have two breasts again. But a lot of the time it doesn't bother me. There are times when...it's really funny because I never really had a cleavage, but there would be times when I'd think it would be nice to look down and have a cleavage. I mean it does change what clothes you wear. I have started to ignore my underarm here and started wearing sleeveless dresses. But I don't wear singlets any more or...I wore a shirt to work the other day and I suppose it was open to about there [pointing], and every time I looked around this lump of plastic was there. So there are little things like that. I won't confront you completely but see I have got the breast there but there's nothing but ribs here. And ok most people don't notice this but other women do. And I don't know. Women are tougher on women than anyone else. So I can only say I suppose it's an emotion thing. It depends on whether I am feeling up or down or, you know, it just depends what is going on and what the situation is.

Jacqui's description of her feelings towards her post-surgical body is illustrative of the complexity of her experience. Her experience is not a singular linear model but is multiple. Pointing to this multiplicity allows Jacqui the freedom to move between seemingly contradictory statements. However, when she feels down she does think about having her breast reconstructed:

I think for some women it [getting a reconstruction] is more important than it is for me. I mean it is something that goes through my head and then when I think about it I'll look through the books and I have seen pictures and I think, I don't know about this. And I have seen one woman and she has got really nice boobs but she has got this revolting scar right across here [pointing to her stomach]. And I thought well if I still want to ride the bike and I still want to do gym, that is really undermining your other tissue. I haven't been doing much lately. But normally. And she's still got the scar across the breast of course. But that was very important to her and to her it was worth it. It's about four operations, four microsurgery. And it's just not that important to me, not that 'whole woman' business.

Just as Jacqui's feelings towards her post-surgical body are multiple, so are her thoughts towards getting a reconstruction. Her experience of other women with 'really nice boobs' but 'revolting scars' is enough to deter her from thinking about it too seriously. She situates herself as different from the women who get it because it is 'not as important' to her. What she articulates as not being as important is 'that "whole woman" business'. She alludes to a very powerful discourse that women use when talking about their post-surgical bodies: that they are not 'complete' or 'whole' after their mastectomy. As a metaphor of recovery, wanting to be 'whole' frames women's post-surgical bodies as incapable of being accepted as normal or natural without two breasts and distances women from the reality of their body.

> I'm still me whether I have one breast, two breasts, or even if I had three. I'm still me. Yes, it would be nice to have two breasts so that I could just stick on a shirt and not worry about having a lump and a hole. You know, I am like everybody else, I like to look nice.

Jacqui refers to the pragmatic aspects of the post-mastectomy body – having to constantly tend to it in order to 'look nice'. She describes herself as happy with who she is, and that the mastectomy has not affected her identity as a woman. However, she feels pressure to cover her 'lump and a hole' and align her appearance with hegemonic norms of femininity.

> I was just pushing myself to get one [a prosthesis]. Because it took me a while to accept that yes I have only got one breast. It's six years now, I have had a lot of practice. But then it was important that I actually get one to fit me. And I had a lot of trouble getting one to fit me. Because I'm a peculiar shape. And even my left breast, the breast tissue is still very firm. I mean it's most unusual for a woman of my age. And most of the shapes are for older women as far as . . . they are more like older women's breasts. Mine has very dense tissue and is hard to match.

In keeping with her survivors attitude Jacqui pushes herself to get a prosthesis. Not having children and being very fit for her age, Jacqui's post-surgical body is difficult to 'fit' for a prosthesis.

> I mean, as I said, after about six weeks when I actually turned around and looked at myself, and I thought, 'well it's not too bad, that's the way it is'. And that's when I started accepting it. And yet like most things it's really up and down. There are times when I think, yes, it would be better if I had two breasts. And then I just get quite defiant and I go swimming without my prosthesis. I am more concerned

about the weight I have put on. But I've just about accepted that. I guess a lot of my attitudes have changed. I am thoroughly enjoying work for the first time for a long time at the moment. But I resign on Monday. And it's been a long time coming but my gut says, you can't keep on going like this.

Jacqui is matter of fact in the way she talks about her post-surgical body, she maintains her strong survivor's attitude and exception from the crowd in describing her defiance in not wearing a prosthesis swimming. Her emphasis on the multiplicity of her feelings about her mastectomized body reveals the instability of this defiance. This instability creates a tension between her body and self and emerges in her work environment as she loses control and gets depression:

Like I have got really high stress tolerance and I just kept pushing it. And of course in the end got pneumonia and thought, oh, I will be back at work in a week. And the doctor said, no you won't. So I ended up having three-and-a-half months off. So it was an accumulation. Like I had been dealing with the cancer bit all last year and that was nine years. You know tumour after tumour. Well, that's over get on with it. And I suppose last year was the crucial year, the five year mark. And I got to the five year mark without any tumours after nine years. And I think just psychologically I started to pack it in. Okay, that's enough, I have made it. Now I can fall apart. And that's how it happened.

She kept 'pushing it', and kept trying to 'get on with it'. This is a constant theme in Jacqui's narrative. Reaching the five-year mark which legitimates status as a survivor has a powerful psychological impact as she starts to 'pack it in' and becomes depressed. She talks about being a survivor:

And even having survived breast cancer there are times when I feel guilty about it. Like I don't have any children, I don't have a husband...Well women are dying of it and they are leaving young families and things like that, whereas if I died there wouldn't be that...okay, there would be family and friends and brothers and sisters, but their daily lives are not affected by my not being there. Whereas women who have children still living at home, some of them very young children, their daily lives. But over the last six months I have actually started working on that and started looking at it and thinking, it's in the lap of the Gods. I survived, I have worked hard to survive. And I have got a survivor's attitude. And a lot of them don't have a survivor's attitude. Yes, I think there is a mixture of fate and control that we have over our lives.

Although Jacqui constantly strived to reach survivorship status, she comments that now she has 'made it' it is something about which she feels guilty. In her narrative both fatalism and self-determination have a role in Jacqui's survival. Although she situates herself as ultimately responsible for it, survivorship signals a point of coherence.

I think more than ever now I live more for the day and I don't take as much life for granted any more. But then I don't wallow in being alive. I am living. Some people will say, but every minute is precious, and I don't sort of consciously think about every minute is precious. That's too much pressure. There is a certain amount of living in being unhappy. It is not real to be happy all the time. What are you hiding from? I mean anguish and mourning and when you go through having a mastectomy that is what you are doing. You are mourning, you are grieving, you have lost a part of yourself. A section of yourself. So there is the anger and the denial. And when you look at yourself there's not much point in denying it...but you still go through all those emotions.

The main theme of Jacqui's narrative is looking to the future but in this last part she contrasts the self she has emphasized as now being one that lives day by day, a perhaps more realistic self. She reveals a softer self, who has been affected by the mastectomy, saying it was a part of who she was. This lies in contrast to the self she refers to earlier as 'still me' with or without breasts. Jacqui is happy with who she is and has accepted her post-surgical body, however, she feels she must wear a prosthesis – the 'lump of plastic' – in order to look nice. Her account reveals that the acceptance of her mastectomized body is unstable and conditional upon a sense of self that is 'up'.

The description of her post-surgical body makes reference to popular psychology notions of identity and breast loss saying 'it's an emotion thing'. Although Jacqui distances herself from 'that "whole woman" business' she is aware of its implications. In saying this she makes an explicit reference to breast cancer discourse that links breast loss to a loss of femininity and identity. She is dismissive of this reference; however, she does consider breast reconstruction from time to time.

This is perhaps linked more to the ambiguity and multiplicity of relating to her post-surgical body than any real need to have her breast reconstructed.

Her narrative relies heavily on discourse of survival and her illness experience is articulated using such tropes as 'getting on with it', 'fighting not to lose' her breast, 'battling and coping', she describes having a 'survivors attitude' and having 'worked hard to survive'. Jacqui positions herself as a battler, constantly trying to move on but repeatedly betrayed by her body as she gets tumour after tumour.

The positive-thinking approach to cancer has been well documented in psycho oncology literature supporting the idea that patients' adjustment to a cancer diagnosis may affect progression of the disease.[20] Positive thinking can be seen as part of the discourse of survival which dominates a lot of mainstream publicity on breast cancer. Fosket *et al.* argue that this produces an insistence on personal responsibility for health and disease. This approach 'reinforces the idea that positive thinking and optimism are far more appropriate responses to illness than are complaint, anger or fear' (2000: 317).

The need to identify as a breast cancer 'survivor' is readily identifiable in women's narratives. Being a survivor carries a certain status that they have 'made it', they have fought and succeeded their 'battle' against disease. In medical terms being a 'breast cancer survivor' means you have lived free of cancer for five years since treatment for breast cancer was labeled a success, even though it does not necessarily mean cancer cannot reoccur after this point. For Jacqui, the recurrences mean she is relegated back to the sick role and again begins the climb to recovery. The images and metaphors she uses indicate a constant strive to normalize her life.

Conclusion

Nell, Rita and Jacqui all experience breast cancer in different contexts and their breast cancer is constructed as different things. For Nell, breast cancer is a relief after 30 years of potential illness, living with the risk of her genetic predisposition 'exploding'. Breast cancer is something she has waited for and expected and was well prepared to deal with. For Nell cancer is located within her body both as she takes on an 'at-risk' identity and also as something which she could have contributed to through various reproductive choices.

Rita's illness takes place in a context of a personal life history of pain and suffering stemming from years of physical and emotional stress. For her, breast cancer is the culmination of years of distress on her self and body and cannot be separated from it. As she articulates, her dealing with the breast cancer is tied up with all these other things in her past. She is not surprised by her diagnosis as she believes the years of abuse have meant a compromised immune system, it is just another assault on her sense of self.

Jacqui's experience of breast cancer occurs over a period of nine years 'tumour after tumour'. She is constantly trying to 'get on with it', to get over the cancer and get on with life. This nine-year 'battle' means that once she does reach five years past her last diagnosis she starts to 'psychologically pack it in'. Her constant strive for survivorship status has left her depressed and needing to resign from work.

A few feminist scholars have analyzed the construction of breast cancer knowledge. They focus on the influence of biomedically defined experiences of breast cancer and the way they fall short of lived experiences (Fosket, 2000), the limited number of meanings from which women can choose when trying to make sense of their illness experience (Rosenbaum and Roos, 2000) and the historical and cultural contexts in which the construction of breast cancer knowledge occurs (Thorne and Murray, 2000).

Fosket (2000) examines how knowledge about breast cancer constructed by biomedical experts does not rely on lived experiences and can, as a result, contradict lived, emotional and embodied experiences. Fosket argues that biomedical constructions are not objective, rational and unproblematic concepts, rather they are profoundly social and emerge out of the complexities of women's experiences and interpretations.

Rosenbaum and Roos identify three areas of meaning that stand out in women's stories: (1) perceptions of breast cancer as equated with death or, alternatively, as manageable and survivable; (2) treatment for breast cancer as compromising to a woman's identity, femininity and self-worth and (3) breast cancer as an experience that should not be openly discussed (2000: 153). An important facet of their analysis is the acknowledgement of the change-over-time meanings and conceptions can have in one's experience. This situates breast cancer as an ever changing and growing experience. They acknowledge women's awareness of trying to find a balance between competing models. Rosenbaum and Roos argue that 'many find that the models do not adequately capture their own feelings and experiences. However, the pervasive nature of these social models serves to mute expression of the myriad ways women can and do respond to breast cancer' (2000: 178).

In the third study, Thorne and Murray (2000) argue that an appreciation of the historical and cultural contexts in which breast cancer imagery has been constructed helps to explain the confusing array of ideologies that confront contemporary women diagnosed with breast cancer. Thorne and Murray argue that when faced with a breast cancer diagnosis, women are presented with competing messages about breast cancer, and that these sets of images, values and strategies can be linked to historical contexts, as well as today's feminist and activist context. They attempt to locate and interpret many of these understandings, creating an analytic context that may help women find their own meanings in their breast cancer experience.

All three women draw on different discourses to articulate their illness experience but give similar references to broader cultural narratives of the body. Nell uses a discourse of risk and military metaphors, Rita uses discourses of pain, vulnerability and victimhood, and Jacqui's account is located firmly within a discourse of survivorship. What is common is their trust and mistrust of the medical profession and the tension between fate and self-determination. The negotiations that each woman describes highlight persistent ambiguity and uncertainty. Thus the narrative acts as a point of reflexivity for these women striving to order the chaos of breast cancer. Instead, what each woman presents is a story that lacks coherence, filled with contradictions and tensions.

Both Nell and Jacqui position themselves at odds with how they assume they are supposed to feel, and attempt to distance themselves from the collective of women who get breast cancer. Nell is not part of the 'sausage factory' emanating fear that she describes, instead she is happy, gay, upbeat and full of relief which she thinks some may find obscene. In addition she sets herself apart from others for whom the loss of a breast is a problem, stating she does not care what others think. Similarly, Jacqui distinguishes herself from the other women for whom body image is a problem: 'it may be important to most women, but not me'. She makes reference to the 'whole woman business', a discourse that does not fit her experience.

All three women articulate confidence in intuitive knowledge of their bodies. Nell articulates that she 'just knew' when she had breast cancer and that she will know before any specialist if she has secondaries. Similarly Rita's reaction to the treatment alerts her that there is something not right about her oncologist's recommendations. She trusts her body to tell her what is wrong. Jacqui also describes faith in her body when her body 'tells' her there is something wrong before she is diagnosed. They all describe an intimate relationship with their body that gives them a sixth sense when something is not quite right. For Nell and Rita, being taken more seriously by their doctors could have made the difference in avoiding certain negative outcomes all together. Instead their knowledge was dismissed as illegitimate kinds of knowing.[21]

At the same time their illness experience creates a disconnection between their body and self. Nell cannot feel normal or natural without her prosthesis, Rita finds her site of surgery unpleasant and her breasts are a site of uncertainty and anxiety as she keeps getting more lumps. Although Jacqui feels comfortable with her mastectomy and will show anyone who wants to look, the way she describes her mastectomy and remaining breast as a 'lump and a hole' is at odds with the symbols of sexuality and nurturing she describes earlier. This self/body dualism has been explored by scholars interested in other facets of women's health.

Research into the sociology and psychology of anorexia nervosa highlights the way anorectics distinguish between the body as it is presented to others (outer body) and the body as it experienced by the anorectic (inner body).[22] Without a connection between the two, a woman cannot come to a new awareness and acceptance of the real state of her corporeality. Garrett argues that people who have fully recovered from anorexia offer the hope that it is possible to abandon an emphasis on the 'ideal body' (the body for others) in favour of the 'felt body' (1997: 145). She suggests that recovery is thus a form of resistance to the self-objectification demanded in our culture. For the mastectomized woman there is quite often a stark distinction between the ideal 'body for others' and the 'felt body', with the 'outer' being a two-breasted pretense filled out with prostheses and the 'inner' a body maimed by breast cancer surgery.

Anorectics talk about a fragmented body and self where there is an anorexic body/mind and inner/outer split.[23] Garrett's respondents spoke of being a 'whole person' indicating a harmony between body and mind. A common thread throughout all of the interviews in my research was women's articulation of wanting to feel 'whole again' following mastectomy. While anorectics use metaphors to describe the 'inner' and the 'outer' body, for mastectomized women 'becoming whole' is a metaphor for recovery where self and body are in harmony. These spatial metaphors simultaneously construct identity as being inside and outside the body. Garrett's (1997) and Malson's (1998) analyses of the distinction between self and body that anorectics articulate is useful for thinking about the disconnection of body and self described by mastectomized women. In the context of this study women describe a disconnection between the self they knew prior to illness, the self they project to others following breast loss and the self they feel they conceal through use of prostheses. Similarly, they have a body 'for others' and a private 'inner' body. Manderson (1999) talks about the need for body harmony in her work on the post-surgical body. Here she suggests that recovery from illness and surgery which leaves changes to the body requires a reclaiming of normalcy.

The removal of a breast brings with it challenges to a woman's sense of femininity.[24] In my interview data femininity is constituted as something superficial. It is about *looking* nice. Women spoke of wanting to feel 'complete' and 'feminine' and saw achieving this as necessitating either the wearing of prostheses or having a breast reconstruction. In doing so the body *appears* whole though underneath it is not. The changed landscape of the mastectomized body means women are forced to redefine themselves as both gendered and sexual despite the absence of a breast or breasts.[25] In not accepting these changes women deny the materiality of their lived bodies. For most women being whole and feminine is constructed in appearance, in the projected ideal body. Quite often this acts to emphasize to the woman the disconnection of body and self as they feel they are withholding the 'truth' about their *real* body.

For Nell, Rita and Jacqui their post-surgical bodies create a tension for their sense of self, of who they are and what lies ahead. The threat to a constituted identity that cancer brings and the subsequent renegotiation of that identity has been explored by many scholars. Mathieson and Stam refer to a 'disrupted feeling of fit' to describe changes from 'the healthy body that one took for granted ... [to the] ill body, under attack from chemotherapeutic agents and the disease itself' (1995: 295). According to Mathieson and Stam negotiating and elaborating the meanings of these changes is part of the 'identity work' facing the patient. Such work necessitates the re-evaluation of meanings upon which the non-ill person based her life,[26] individual dealings with the stigma of cancer[27] and the patient's voice as it exists amongst the constraints of the discourse of medicine.[28] All of these negotiations impact on the ways in which the sick and healthy body dwell in often uncomfortable and paradoxical relation to each other.[29]

Both Nell and Rita have required constant medical surveillance and as a result risk is experienced as a condition of 'non-health', transformed into a symptom of a future illness.[30] Being classified as 'at risk' necessitates an embodiment of an 'at-risk' identity.[31] For Nell an identity shift takes place as her genetic history is realized and the inevitable cancer removed through bilateral mastectomy. For Rita an identity struggle emerges when a state of perpetual 'non-health' goes unresolved. Nell and Rita have similarly experienced tensions when trying to identify with the sick role.

According to Parsons (1951) identifying with this role necessitates four things: social withdrawal from certain obligations such as work and family duties; exemption from responsibility for their medical condition; accepting the social obligation to improve and get better and seeking out professional medical expertise. Although Parsons's contribution to medical sociology has been criticized,[32] it is useful to discuss the strains in women's narratives regarding being legitimately 'well' or 'sick', and the ambiguous state some women are in, when caught between these two socially defined roles.

Nell reiterates that she does not feel disfigured but in order to re-establish a sense of normality and feeling sexy she must wear prostheses. She wants to make the statement that not wearing a prosthesis makes that she accepts her body the way it is, but is caught in a bind between what being sexy and nice means. The consequence of Rita choosing a quadrantectomy instead of a mastectomy means she is never situated as fully recovered, she is caught in a space between ill and well and cannot gain legitimate status in either. Her post-surgical body is one of ambiguity and anxiety. Although Jacqui feels quite comfortable with her post-surgical body she thinks about reconstruction often. While ultimately she does not think all the extra surgery is worth it, looking down and seeing a 'lump of plastic' and sometimes feeling as though she would like a cleavage lead her to reconsider. She describes this as an 'emotion thing', sometimes feeling ok about her body and sometimes not. What Jacqui alludes to is the multiplicity of her experience; however, when she is not feeling ok about her body she feels her only option is to get a reconstruction. For Jacqui, just like Nell and Rita there seems to be no other mechanisms available through which to regain a sense of normalcy.

As I go on to show in the following chapters, a major locus of trying to find coherence in practice is in how women perform their post-surgical bodies in everyday life. Much of the work that examines the post-surgical body after breast cancer constructs the mastectomized body as essentially lacking and in need of being 'restored' to how it *looked* prior to surgery.[33] This study identifies and challenges the lack of positive discourse on the post-surgical body. A notable silence permeates women's narratives and casts the mastectomized body as *other*.

Nell, Rita and Jacqui all draw from a range of readily available scripts to discuss their diverse illness experiences. However, no alternative scripts exist for talking about the post-surgical body. Instead the only narrative available locates recovery from breast loss as necessitating recovering two breasts. What is offered to women is the choice of either wearing a prosthesis or having a reconstruction, both of which I go on to show have limited value in reconstructing the sense of self that is deeply challenged during the breast cancer experience.

3
Pink Advocacy: Camaraderie, Competition and the Making of a Breast Cancer Career

Introduction

The lights go down, and we sit momentarily in silence. Then, Boom, Boom, Boom, music thumps from enormous speakers at every corner of the room and overhead. 'It's a Beautiful Life', the theme song for tonight's Annual Bosom Buddies Fashion Parade is almost deafening. Spotlights swirl onto the stage and a dozen women clad in their hot pink Bosom Buddies t-shirts and long black pants come skipping (dancing?) out on stage. One by one they do a lap of the cat walk, waving, clapping, smiling, singing. The audience joins in the rhythmic applause and the 'models' assemble on stage holding hands, beaming. The music is lowered and the organizer of tonight's gala event, Barbara, exclaims 'Wasn't that fantastic!' Another round of ecstatic applause from the crowd. The models scurry behind the curtain and the music is gone. Barbara takes a more sombre tone and sincerely thanks the wife of a doctor who has come tonight on behalf of, it seems, the entire medical establishment. Barbara also thanks any other medical professionals who may be unidentified in the audience. The Bosom Buddies mission statement is read out and Barbara invites all those women in the audience who have breast cancer or who are survivors to stand up. Again, deafening applause.

Enter stage left, the celebrity compare head to toe in flushing pink. Tina, an actress whose portfolio includes leading guest roles in 'A Country Practice' and 'Flying Doctors', takes the microphone and expresses that 'all of you here take a very special place in my heart'. She then gives her breast cancer story, complete with tales of liaising with a 'famous' gynecologist. 'There is life after breast cancer' she gushes, 'God Bless'.

The song 'I will survive' thuds from the speakers and lights bounce off the glittering pink sashes that border the stage: 'Ladies and Gentlemen...Daywear!'. The models skip out on stage one by one, their hair and makeup reminiscent of a debutante ball. Tina draws our attention to the 'cute' shorts, 'yummy' tops and 'delicious' colours being modeled as the women play out their clunky choreographed routine. 'Next up...Swimwear!' shouts Tina and oohs and aahs rise from the crowd. Out they come bouncing oversized inflatable beach balls to one another, their rigid smiles masking any anxiety of parading in their bathers. Most wear large unbuttoned shirts over the top but one woman models just a bikini to which there is even greater applause. The compare drawls: 'Don't the girls look gorrgeeous!'...

Bosom Buddies, the force behind this gala event, is one of many breast cancer support and advocacy groups in Australia. The night raises thousands of dollars for medical research and the women involved declare loudly how happy they are with their second chance at life. However, amongst the glitz and glamour of the evening one thing remains hidden – the mastectomized body. Women parade their restored two-breasted bodies, illustrating succinctly that a 'celebration of life' is not complete without a restoration of two breasts. The post-surgical body in mainstream breast cancer culture is by and large shrouded in secrecy, something to be covered up and not spoken about.

Primarily a fundraising and advocacy organization, Bosom Buddies have no set office, paid staff or fixed meeting room. The organization is made up of a committee of six volunteers and over 300 members from Canberra and surrounding regions. Members meet monthly to discuss upcoming fundraising events and pass on the latest fundraising ideas. Their quarterly newsletter covers latest research findings, local fundraising events, summaries of conferences members have attended and stories and poems from readers. Founded in 1993, Bosom Buddies mission is 'to provide a service to those living with breast cancer and their families through support, advocacy and training' (Bosom Buddies, 2003a). They endorse the local 'Look good...Feel better' (LGFB) programme, a cosmetics workshop run at the Canberra Hospital (sponsored by various member companies of the Cosmetic, Toiletry and Fragrance Association (CTFA) of Australia) for women being treated for cancer, and fund and promote 'Caring for You', a mobile post-mastectomy prosthesis and lingerie business. They have developed a telephone counseling service where newly diagnosed women can phone and speak to a Bosom Buddies volunteer who has had similar treatment and surgery. In addition, Bosom Buddies members do rounds of hospitals handing out information packages to breast cancer patients and acting as a first point of contact in the breast cancer community.

With 'sister' organizations in both the United States and the United Kingdom, Bosom Buddies is representative of grass-roots advocacy and fundraising groups who perpetuate a mainstream breast cancer culture, and whose aim is to support 'salvationist science, surveillance medicine and individual vigilance' and thrust survivorship identities and heteronormative femininities into the foreground (Klawiter, 2000: 87).

In *The Cancer Journals* (1980), Audre Lorde, a black lesbian feminist poet, describes her experience of breast cancer. Shortly after waking from her operation, Lorde is visited by a woman from 'Reach for Recovery', an American version of the Bosom Buddies volunteer programme. The woman, like her Australian counterparts, comes equipped with a temporary prosthesis to give the newly mastectomized woman. Lorde finds herself staring in the mirror at the prosthesis she has just put in her bra – 'perched on my chest askew, awkwardly inert and lifeless, and having nothing to do with any me I could possibly conceive of' (1980: 33) – thinking that perhaps the woman from Reach for Recovery knows something she doesn't, that she would feel entirely different once it was on.

> I looked at the large gentle curve my left breast made under the pyjama top. A curve that seemed even larger now that it stood by itself. I looked strange and uneven and peculiar to myself, but somehow, ever so much more myself, and therefore so much more acceptable, than I looked with that thing stuck inside my clothes. For not even the most skilful prosthesis in the world could undo that reality, or feel the way my breast had felt, and either I would love my body one-breasted now, or remain forever alien to myself. (1980: 33)

Usually strong and confident, Lorde emphasizes the sense of vulnerability she felt immediately after her mastectomy:

> [W]ithin this period of quasi-numbness and almost childlike susceptibility to ideas...many patterns and networks are started for women...that encourage us to deny the realities of our bodies which have just been driven home to us so graphically, and these old and stereotyped patterns of response pressure us to reject the adventure and exploration of our own experience, difficult and painful as those experiences may be (1980: 30).

This chapter is concerned with the construction of meanings of the post-surgical body within the breast cancer movement. I argue that mainstream breast cancer culture mobilizes a specific breast cancer identity which promotes aesthetic hegemony and frames the mastect-omized body as unfeminine, abnormal and desexualized. This chapter is also concerned with the politics of this women's health movement. Like any organization, breast cancer support and advocacy groups contain a hierarchy based on certain credentials. In this study women spoke about a social ladder based on the extent of surgery, availability of time and energy and willingness to conform to dominant attitudes and belief systems. I argue that a woman's standing within the breast cancer community can have implications for her eligibility to participate in certain work, such as being a consumer representative. The breast cancer community in Australia is made up of a number of high-profile 'survivors' who have a significant presence on medical, research, and advocacy boards and committees. The micropolitics of such groups has the potential to frame women's experiences negatively and the women who dominate them remain largely unchallenged. Women who question these beliefs or outlooks mostly remain silent or withdraw from the community all together.

Like much of the feminist work that has been done on discourse and identity, this research is concerned with the ways cultural and medical discourses have worked to homogenize and normalize the female body by presenting women with an ideological picture of femininity and insisting that all women aspire to this ideal.[1] I want to pay particular attention to a cultural discourse that is taken for granted by the women involved in breast cancer support and advocacy groups and wider society, as largely feminist and empowering, and reveal it instead to be potentially harmful and restrictive. The discourses embedded within the mainstream breast cancer movement reproduce and promote notions of women's mastectomized bodies as being socially and personally unacceptable.

The breast cancer movement

Whilst the history of the breast cancer movement in Australia is largely unmapped, detailed histories of the movement in Canada[2] and United States[3] provide important insights into how gender and emotions are publicly mobilized and performed,[4] how breast cancer activism discur-sively engages the authorities and priorities of science and medicine[5] and the workings of power within breast cancer groups.[6] For the most part this literature situates the breast cancer movement as an inherently feminist movement, ultimately empowering women and improving their health and quality of life.

The emergence of breast cancer–specific organizations

As early as 1913 cancer organizations had begun to emerge in the United States.[7] These organizations were formed in response to various needs and interests; to facilitate cancer research, to provide the most modern methods for the diagnosis and treatment of cancer, and to raise money from the public to fund research, and patient and carers facilities.

In the early 1950s research from both England and the United States correlating cigarette smoking and lung cancer was being widely reported in the media, and cancer began to appear as a major health issue. Interest in cancer treatment, prevention, and cures began to increase and cancer organizations began to lobby Health Departments to undertake public education about the dangers of smoking. During the early 1970s cancer research and education campaigns focused on getting legislation passed requiring cigarette packets to be labeled with health warnings. At the same time breast cancer–specific support services were also being established. This was in a period of intensive community-based feminist activism that saw the establishment of an abortion referral service and the Leichhardt women's health centre in Sydney in 1974.[8] Breast cancer–specific support services, known as Mastectomy Rehabilitation Services (MRS), were formed in conjunction with state-based cancer organizations.[9]

The MRS program was developed in Australia as an adaptation of the Reach to Recovery program which was started by Therese Lasser in New York in 1952. Lasser persuaded the medical community that it was extremely valuable for a woman diagnosed with breast cancer to have the opportunity to see and talk with a woman who had been in a similar situation who has recovered and returned to normal lifestyle activities.

Reach to Recovery has a global audience with programmes in Australia, the United States, United Kingdom, South Africa and across Europe (more than 70 groups in 50 countries). They have an international website, newsletter 'Bloom', and a conference every three years.[10]

In Australia the MRS was renamed as the Breast Cancer Support Service (BCSS) at the beginning of the 1980s and operates in all states and territories through state cancer organizations affiliated with The Cancer Council.

The principal aim of BCSS is to provide one-on-one emotional support and practical information to people who have breast cancer. Peer support is provided by cancer council–trained volunteers who have experienced breast cancer at least 18 months previously. Volunteers are from a wide age range and a wide diversity of treatments, backgrounds and interests.

Shortly after developing BCSS, another US-born cancer service, LGFB was established in Australia in 1990. LGFB is a free national community service program that aims to teach women cancer patients, through hands-on experience, techniques to help restore their appearance and self-image during chemotherapy and radiation treatment. The program was founded and developed by the CTFA and it is administered through the registered charitable organization, The Cancer Patients Foundation Ltd. LGFB relies on the CTFA and its member companies to provide the makeup, materials and financial support for the program. LGFB also has international appeal with its 'sister' programmes established in Europe, the United Kingdom and South Africa.

The philosophies of both the BCSS and the LGFB had a dominating influence on the development of grass-roots breast cancer support and advocacy groups.

Grass-roots organizations

Breaking away from the traditional cancer council–run support group, the beginnings of Canberra's Bosom Buddies are typical of the more than 100 breast cancer fundraising and support groups around Australia today and thousands across the United Kingdom and America.

The beginnings of Bosom Buddies are typical of the start of many of these grass-roots organizations. In the early 1990s, during her own breast cancer diagnosis and treatment, Shirley Fitzgerald had attended the ACT Cancer Council BCSS on a regular basis and had been doing volunteer work with the community nurses at The Canberra Hospital. Shirley was called upon when a woman presented with breast cancer and needed some support from someone with a similar experience. In 1994, Shirley, and two other women who were having treatment for breast cancer, decided that they needed something different from the support service offered by the cancer council; they sought something that was more social, something that was not as regimented as the BCSS. In Shirley's words, they wanted to be able to laugh. The group started as a small number of women going out for dinner together, or to one another's home's for coffee, where they were free to talk about things other than their breast cancer experience as they felt limited to do at the BCSS.

Shirley had helped run a fashion parade with the ACT Cancer Council and when they no longer wanted to continue with it, Shirley suggested Bosom Buddies to take over. It was from this that awareness and membership of their group grew. With money being raised from the fashion parade they needed to become more formalized, and two years after they began they had a structured committee and developed a mission statement outlining their aims and objectives.

Similar groups that are either extensions of the Cancer Council BCSS or completely independent have since formed in all states and territories in Australia.[11] These groups often have a website and newsletter, and offshoot special interest support groups, for example for younger women, indigenous women or partners.

In the same year that Bosom Buddies formed, a larger state-based advocacy group was established. Similar to the Susan G. Komen Foundation in North America, the Breast Cancer Action Group (BCAG) was the first group of its kind in Australia. It began as a group of women meeting monthly at the home of Marcia O'Keefe, a woman whose experience with breast cancer had led her to be part of a working party putting together the first clinical practice guidelines for the treatment of early breast cancer (drafted by the National Health and Medical Research Council (NH&MRC) and taken over by the NBCC when it was set up in 1995). Shortly after joining this national working party, she was invited to join the Consumer Advisory Committee of BreastScreen Victoria, of which she became Chair. A BCAG newsletter, marking the tenth anniversary of the group, noted the difficulty in setting the group up and the 'hard-working women whose fingers were burnt' (2004: 2) when trying to script BCAG's constitution. Marcia was determined it would be a feminist group; however, questions that arose about how issues would be decided, for example by voting, elicited negative responses as 'a feminist approach required consensus, but that took forever' (2004: 2). BCAG's slogan, 'Giving a voice to women with breast cancer', helped ground their approach and they became committed to ensuring that consumer voices were heard. One of the first major contributions by the group was a petition to get the drug Taxol on the Pharmaceutical Benefits Scheme. This petition, which began in Marcia's living room, was later presented in Parliament.

The BCAG New South Wales (NSW) began as a sister organization in 1997 and have published numerous booklets on what to expect after a breast cancer diagnosis, hold information forums for women each year and have recently produced the Directory of Breast Cancer Treatment and Services for NSW Women. In conjunction with BCAG Victoria, they helped start the national level Breast Cancer Network Australia (BCNA).

The National Women's Health Policy and the establishment of national breast cancer organizations

Throughout the 1980s state-based women's health policies were being produced as a result of intensive feminist activism around public policy development and in 1986 a national organization, the Australian Women's Health Network (AWHN), was established by women's health campaigners to involve and represent women in major health-related developments.

In 1989 after a long consultative process with various women's organizations, the National Women's Health Policy was produced, which emphasized a social rather than medical approach to women's health. In regard to breast cancer the policy acknowledged the need for an evaluation of a national screening program, combined with the need to immediately increase public awareness of mammography.[12] The national BreastScreen program was officially launched in 1991.

With statistics denoting the increased incidence of breast cancer in Australia (up by 25% from 1977 to 1990) breast cancer was receiving a great deal of publicity. In addition, the federal government's funding allocations to the disease was in recognition of the importance of the disease as a public health problem, and a sign of its commitment to women's issues.

With BreastScreen Australia underway breast cancer was firmly in the media spotlight. The result was an explosion of breast cancer support and advocacy groups around the country, from small town-based groups to larger-scale, more structured organizations that lobbied government. The mid-1990s also saw the establishment of two national organizations whose purpose is to raise money for scientific research into breast cancer.

The Kathleen Cuningham Foundation, now known as the NBCF, was the result of a $3 million grant from the Labour government in 1994. The NBCF is Australia's only national not-for-profit foundation established to promote and support research into every aspect of breast cancer. With considerable corporate sponsorship and very successful fundraising campaigns (for example, Fashion Targets Breast Cancer, Pink Ribbon Magazine, and the Mother's Day Classic Fun Run), the NBCF is able to offer millions of dollars in research grants focused primarily on scientific projects. International comparisons include the Susan G. Komen Foundation and the NBCF (USA) and Breast Cancer Care (UK), who also receive large corporate sponsorship and, on a much larger scale, run similarly themed fundraising campaigns.

The NBCC was established in 1995 by the Australian Government in response to community concerns about the human cost of breast cancer. (In 1999 the Government provided funding to expand their work into ovarian cancer.) The NBCC claims that they work from the assumption that mortality and morbidity from breast cancer can be significantly improved if the knowledge gained from health research is better translated into practice. As CEO of the NBCC, Christine Ewan argued that since its formation the organization has developed a systematic and evidence-based approach to improving care by demonstrating a need for change, careful analysis and trialing of innovative strategies to improve formation, practice and policy. They have consumer representatives involved on all of their advisory groups and working parties.

The NBCC has a large focus on public education campaigns to help raise community awareness about a range of breast and ovarian cancer issues. In addition they develop national surveys to help gauge community perceptions and behavior in relation to breast and ovarian cancer so as to better understand and respond to community needs.

From the outset the NBCC worked closely with emerging consumer organizations and established a national consumer advisory group to provide advice on its programs. One of the initiatives of this group was a national meeting for breast cancer advocates in Canberra, which over 300 women attended. It also resulted in the establishment of the BCNA. Consumers made a major contribution to the development of the NBCC. They had a key role in agenda setting, raising the importance of many issues such as travel and accommodation, breast nurses, young women with breast cancer and breast reconstruction. Lymphodema was an issue of particular concern; it was almost entirely as a result of advocacy by consumers that a national meeting was held in Adelaide to establish a research agenda to improve understanding of lymphodema.

The BCNA was officially launched at the inaugural of *Field of Women* in Canberra in October 1998, following the First National Breast Cancer Conference for Women. BCNA is funded through donations from the community, corporate sponsorship and fundraising events and has also received grants from Commonwealth and State government departments to assist specific projects. One of the aims of the BCNA is to be a national umbrella body capable of combining groups such as BCAG and other similar groups that were forming, into one strong national voice. BCNA has state representatives in each state and territory. The role of the state reps is to recruit and liaise with member groups and individuals, promote the BCNA's role and activities within their own state, respond to 'calls for action' from the National office and organize such things as public forums within their own state. Ninety-seven groups make up the BCNA's members[13] and include BCAG Victoria and NSW, Bosom Buddies, numerous Cancer Council Support Groups and Lymphodema support groups.

Some of the well-known advocacy and fundraising events include the BCNA's 'Field of Women' and the NBCF's 'Bras Across the Bridge'. The Field of Women began in 1998 and involves the display of thousands of identical pink silhouettes on the lawns of Parliament House in Canberra, and other prominent sites across Australia, representing the number of women diagnosed with breast cancer each year. This event promotes breast cancer awareness month and the BCNA and is meant to depict a 'graphic display of breast cancer statistics' (BCNA, 2001). In a mass symbol of aesthetic hegemony, these silhouettes resemble large-scale paper dolls and make no secret of the feminine theme of breast cancer culture. The hyperfeminine symbol depicts the female body clad in an a-line dress, legs and heels together with feet pointed outwards and bobbed hair that flicks out at the ends. The arms sit outward from the torso, cut off at the elbows.

'Bras Across the Bridge' is held annually by the NBCF in conjunction with local Sydney radio station 2Day FM. In 2002, 900 bras were strung across Pyrmont Bridge at Darling Harbour, and 2Day FM listeners pledged a donation per bra. Volunteers on the bridge sold pink ribbons to drivers and all proceeds went to 'research'. The dominant feminine theme of breast cancer culture that these two events promote is also reflected in the media's portrayal of the disease and the women it affects.

Activities of the BCNA have included the annual Field of Women and the A Seat at the Table Program (described later in chapter), the lobbying for the drug Herceptin to be available free of cost to women with advanced breast cancer, the presentation of the 'Warrior Women' multimedia traveling exhibition and the production of the 'My Journey' information kit for women diagnosed with breast cancer. In 2002 they had 7600 members and nine staff.

The breast cancer movement has its roots in the women's health movement of the 1970s and 1980s when women fought to change their relation to medical institutions, practitioners and knowledges.[14] Kaufert (1998) argues that since then women with breast cancer have 'gradually put together an oppositional discourse in which they have reinterpreted the meaning of being a woman with cancer, challenged existing stereo-types of how they should behave, and demanded recognition of a new paradigm' (1998: 288). According to Kaufert, this has grown from a focus on the individual encounter to a more macrolevel, insisting on an overhaul of the relationship between women and the medical and research profession (1998: 288).

Whilst certain tropes of feminism have informed the breast cancer movement, and examples of activism which do promote diversity within the breast cancer community exist[15] there is little evidence of such an overhaul in the mainstream of breast cancer culture today. Instead women are saturated in feminine themed colours and fund-raising for medical and scientific causes with celebrity breast cancer 'ambassadors'. The Bosom Buddies fashion parade encompasses what Barbara Ehrenreich describes as the 'cult of pink kitsch' that drenches much mainstream breast cancer culture (2001: 43).

Breast cancer in the media

In the last few years there has been a proliferation of information about breast cancer in the popular media. The media has been used as an effective tool to raise awareness of the disease and promote the need for funding. However, questions that feminists have raised about the expanding profile of breast cancer in the media are what types of know-ledge are being produced and what are the effects of that knowledge production?[16]

Reviews of breast cancer in the media have identified strong associations between the disease and issues of femininity.[17] The linking of risk for breast cancer with reproductive choices is one such correlation.[18] Deborah Lupton finds that the messages conveyed in many Australian news articles suggest that 'women who refused to adopt the traditional feminine maternal role...were courting disaster' (1994b: 75). She suggests that the overt content of press accounts are underpinned by subtle messages regarding women's role in society, women's bodies, and the nature of femininity.

Saywell *et al.* (2000) suggest that the iconography of breast cancer is structured by images of the fetishized and idealized youthful breast. Their analysis of press coverage in the United Kingdom demonstrates that the 'sexiness' of breasts is used to 'sell' breast cancer and, corre-spondingly, mastectomies are constructed as a violation of femininity. Saywell *et al.* argue that while the 'cancerous' breast can be neither erotic nor maternal, it is constantly situated in relation to either or both of these dominant discourses of femininity. Like other forms of ampu-tation, the authors suggest that 'perceptions of mastectomy and lumpectomy are governed by ideas about disfigurement, damage and mutilation' (2000: 43), their association being with disease and not recovery.

With press coverage focusing largely on young, attractive women's accounts of breast cancer, even more attention is given to the asymmetry of mastectomy and lumpectomy representing an assault on beauty and perceptions of normality. Saywell *et al.* emphasize that the 'processes surrounding mastectomy and post-operative recovery are designed to reaffirm and reproduce sexual and gender identities' (2000: 43). Stacey argues, 'to keep one's femininity intact requires elaborate efforts on the part of the woman with cancer: above all, energy should be directed into covering up the signs of this stigmatized disease and the effects of its treatments' (1997: 71). Alternative media, such as activist photography have openly and beautifully portrayed women's post-mastectomy body, reconfiguring the post-surgical female body in public space.

In 1991 the artist and model Matuschka was diagnosed with breast cancer and had a mastectomy. Following her surgery, which she discovered had not been necessary, Matuschka became an activist on breast cancer issues. Hoping to increase awareness of the prevalence of breast cancer and also to suggest a more positive self-image for women who had had mastectomies, she continued producing artistic portraits of herself, many of them revealing the results of her mastectomy.

Her career took a very public turn with the appearance of her photographic self-portrait on the cover of the *New York Times Magazine* on 15 August, 1993. (She appears in a tailored white dress cut away from her right shoulder and torso to give a full view of her mastectomy scar.) This photo titled 'Beauty Out of Damage' was accompanied by Susan Ferraro's article, 'The Anguished Politics of Breast Cancer'. In an interview with *Glamour Magazine* (November 1993) explaining her motivation for the NYT photo Matuschka comments:

> Are women that vain? I refuse to believe that the majority of us value our lives less than our breasts. That we would rather live in fear or get sick and die than take simple preventative measures. I have always adhered to the philosophy that one should speak and show the truth, because knowledge leads to free will, to choice. If we keep quiet about what breast cancer does to women's bodies, if we refuse to accept women's bodies in whatever condition they are in, we are doing a disservice to womankind ... My picture was about the choice made by me and many other women: We decided not to subject ourselves to any more reconstructive surgery, with all its risks, not to go through any more deceptions about our appearance and the risks to well-being that they can create.

Matuschka has taken a strong stand against reconstructive surgery and the use of prostheses, because, she says, as an artist she prefers the difficult truth to the social lie that denies the difficult reality of cancer and breast removal.

Another breast cancer artist and activist, Jo Spence, provides a powerful series of self-portrait photographs documenting the artist's fight against breast cancer, accompanied by a narrative describing her responses to the medical community.[19]

In Australia the Warrior Women Exhibition, an initiative of the BCNA, invited women of all ages, cultural and social backgrounds, to collaborate with women artists to develop responses to their own experience with breast cancer. The collaborations took place over a two-year period and resulted in over 100 pieces of mixed media art which were shown around Australia in 2002.

At these sites breast cancer 'becomes a crucial site for the re-evaluation of what counts as a beautiful body, and what meaning age, race and cultural identity have in a culture where disease and health technologies are reconstructing what a healthy body is, and what particular body parts mean'.[20]

The heteronormative femininity promoted by the breast cancer movement in Australia is not limited to fundraising events. Pink advocacy has taken on wider currency mobilized in an annual national magazine, *Pink Ribbon*. Launched in 2002 the magazine is produced by the NBCF and the editorial board of *Marie Clare* magazine and captures the essence of mainstream breast cancer culture.

Pretty in pink

At a glance *Pink Ribbon* is like any other glossy women's magazine on the market. Sold in newsagents across the country it features celebrities, fashion, and beauty tips. However, for a magazine that by all appearances looks like others marketed to the 18–30-age bracket, sex is notably absent. Along with the soft pink hues which emanate from the glossy magazine are messages about women's health and beauty and the post-surgical body. Through infantilising and feminising tropes the woman with breast cancer is constructed as ultra-feminine and desexualized and the mastectomized body as one that is at best temporary and at worst able to be hidden.

Saturated in soft pink pastel, the inside cover of the 2002 edition features a double-page advertisement for Estee Lauder 'Pink Ribbon' lip gloss. The advertisement urges women to 'join the crusade' against breast cancer by purchasing their product, proceeds of which go to an undisclosed charity. The following page is an advertisement for the David Jones Charity Bear. 'Theodore' the brown plush teddy (complete with pink ribbon) is a 'cuddly, handsome gift for both children and adults'. A couple of pages later is an advertisement for a Baume & Mercier watch with interchangeable hot pink strap. Other pink breast cancer–themed products which feature in the magazine include 'Pink Pocket Equal' artificial sweetener tablets, pink 'pearls of hope' from Michael Hill jewellers, limited edition pink-tubbed Meadow Lea margarine, Harlequin Mills and Boon 'Pink Ribbon' titles and Hallmark 'pink ribbon' Christmas cards. There is also a special 'In the Pink' fashion spread on must have accessories, from pink high heels and bikini to pink candles and wine glasses.

The articles are mostly sickly sweet features: 'The feel-good calendar', 'Thanks for the mammaries', '50 things to make you smile' (some examples include puppies, babies, rose petals, rubber ducks, love heart candy, knitted dolls, frothy cappuccinos, 'playing footsy', rosy-cheeked garden gnomes, ribbons and bows and sand castles), 'Friends: celebrities and their best mates', 'Pink inspiration: Photographers look through rose-tinted lenses', 'Look good, feel great: If we have to look sensational in order to feel fabulous then who are we to fight it?' and so on. Even those focusing on more serious issues such as funding for 'science' (bordered in pink-tinted blood cells) and advice on reducing risk use overly simplistic repertoire to relay information: 'Drinking 2 litres of water a day will make you look and feel better, but . . . although it has a cute medical name – polydipsia – drinking large amounts of water is dangerous' (2002: 104).

Barbara Ehrenreich (2001) argues that the use of infantilising tropes in breast cancer culture suggests that perhaps 'regression to a state of childlike dependency puts one in the best frame of mind with which to endure the prolonged and toxic treatments' or alternatively that 'femininity is by its nature incompatible with full adulthood – a state of arrested development' (2001: 46). This could possibly account for the absence of sex in an otherwise 'normal' women's magazine of the same genre. Alternatively, the emphasis on 'looking good' (by restoring breast shape) is not for the benefit of a (most probably) male partner, but to 'show off to the girls' (2002: 30). Personal stories from breast cancer survivors situate the mastectomized body as 'ugly without any clothes on' (2002: 24) and 'ugly, ugly, ugly' (2002: 30). Indeed, the magazine contains no positive images of the mastectomized post-surgical body at all.

Staying positive

A common thread throughout all facets of the breast cancer movement is the promotion of an 'upbeat image' which focuses on prevention, early detection and survivorship, not death.[21] Advocacy and support groups, like Bosom Buddies, work hard at getting their message across. However, what is at issue is exactly what that message is. Celia Roberts argues that:

> [W]hilst it could be seen as feminist to simply educate women about the science of breast cancer, to encourage women to tell their stories, and to teach women the skills of advocacy...women involved with breast cancer should go further...Women's health issues are not about toeing the medical line, or getting more money spent on women's diseases, or being allowed to sit quietly on decision-making committees. Rather, women's health issues, such as breast cancer, are political issues. They concern the ways in which medical and scientific knowledge and practices produce women's bodies differently to men's. (2000:5)

Within Australian breast cancer culture there is little discussion of differences between women and of the need for the development of skills recognizing that women are diverse, and have varying interests and needs. As Batt (1994) argues, advocates need to be careful not to participate in situations where they actually contribute (through lack of awareness) to the oppression of certain groups of women. This has occurred, for example, in the area of breast cancer support services – in the United States, Canada and Australia – where lesbian women have been discriminated against by other breast cancer survivors' narrow views of 'acceptable' feminine behaviors and appearance. Audre Lorde gives a moving and angry description of her experiences in the 1970s in the United States when she was criticized by a support volunteer worker for failing to wear a prosthesis.[22] This volunteer was unable to respond sensitively to Lorde's desires to talk about integrating breast cancer into her life (a life that did not involve trying to 'catch a man' or concerns about embarrassing her children in front of their friends). In research commissioned by the NBCC in Australia, Kissane *et al.* (1999) found similarly that lesbian women with breast cancer did not feel comfortable revealing their sexual preferences to BCSS volunteers.

In line with what Klawiter (2000) describes of certain aspects of American breast cancer culture, the 'culture of action' in Australia mobilizes and promotes the 'heterofeminine, resilient body: the repaired, reconstructed body beautiful'.[23] At this level femininity is discursively mediated through women's experiences. According to Smith, women actively 'do femininity': 'Women are not just the passive products of socialization; they are active; they create themselves' (1990: 161). Thus femininity is conceptualized in terms of ongoing actual practices of individuals: femininity requires knowing what needs to be done to remedy one's body, assessing the possibilities, and acting upon them.[24] Viewing femininity as a discourse, Smith (1990) argues that women interpret discourse via ideologies and doctrines of femininity which are explicit and publicly spoken and written.

Pink Ribbon and events such as the Bosom Buddies fashion parade depict the post-surgical body as something which must be kept hidden and ultimately corrected. They demand a refiguring of the body to fit the heteronormative ideals of femininity that are so succinctly portrayed in the pink, female symbols of the 'Field of Women'. Such public displays mobilize these norms making it almost impossible to renegotiate an identity outside these heavily promoted stereotypes.

The making of a breast cancer career

The piece de resistance of the evening requires a verbal drum roll from the compare: 'it takes a lot of courage to get up here, I bet you never thought you'd see them like this...Lingerie!'. Negligees and matching bras and underwear are showcased. The crowd applauds incessantly. Each woman wears a shawl draped over her back and arms and there is almost a standing ovation when one woman throws her shawl out into the audience. 'Don't they look pretty!' Tina shouts with glee 'So feminine'. 'Thank you girls' she adds as they exit the stage.

The lights go up as preparation is made for the more serious part of the evening – the 'biographies'. As the models prepare backstage, time is taken to thank each sponsor again. I use the time to peruse the program, thinking I might get a head start on these biographies. Headshots of the twelve models are each accompanied by a few lines of text: Linda Toll, Diagnosed 1998, Lumpectomy, Radical Mastectomy, Chemotherapy, Radiotherapy; Beatrice Rand, Diagnosed 2000, Lumpectomy, Mastectomy, Reconstruction; Cecelia Barton, Diagnosed 1993, Mastectomy, Tamoxifen, and so on.

> *Soft, instrumental music prepares us for the sentimentality of the finale to tonight's 'celebration'. Barbara takes the microphone as a large pink ribbon gains prominence on the screen behind her. The first of the twelve models, Betty, walks slowly across the stage, eyes downcast and hands limp by her side. As she approaches Barbara a large basket of roses is brought up to the stage. Barbara draws one from the bunch and dramatically outstretches her arm to give it to her. Betty clutches the rose, smells it and continues her journey along the catwalk. Her biography is read out detailing when and where she was diagnosed, the extent of her surgery and treatment and her survivorship status. She adds a personal quote from Betty, expressing her gratitude for the doctors who 'put her back together' when she had her breast reconstruction.*
>
> *By the end Betty is sobbing and I brace myself for the next eleven. The biographies are painfully slow and dreadfully sad and I am near tears by the end. All of the models gather on stage, each having had their turn in the limelight. The final point in their choreographed routine sees them simultaneously throw their roses in the air and skip out along the catwalk as 'It's a Beautiful Life' blasts from the speakers for a final time. The crowd cheers, the models look relieved and emotional . . .*

At the Bosom Buddies fashion parade each woman's past and present is neatly packaged into a breast cancer CV, contextualized only in comparison to other women's breast cancer careers. Marital status, age, occupation, children or interests are excluded in place of individual breast cancer demographics. Regardless of who these women were prior to their diagnosis, breast cancer offers a new framing. The renegotiation of identity during and after a breast cancer crisis necessitates re-evaluating the meaning and purpose of their lives and for some involves finding ways to 'give something back' to the breast cancer community.

Equipped with the right expertise – a breast cancer experience – women are qualified to participate in an important component of their new breast cancer self: volunteer work. In programs like that run by Bosom Buddies and Reach for Recovery, where breast cancer survivors visit newly diagnosed patients in hospital, the volunteer is positioned as having authority and expertise and empowered by their experiential knowledge. In addition to giving out an 'attractive bag' to hold post-surgery drainage collection bags, a temporary 'fluffy duck' prosthesis, small heart-shaped cushions which can be placed under the arms for comfort during recovery from surgery, and various information leaflets, volunteers offer their own experiences and advice.

Giving something back

I spoke with women about why they got involved with volunteer work. Maya, 53, is a public servant and a married mother of two adult children.

> The support I thought was something I wanted to do to give back. I knew how much it had meant to me to meet other women with breast cancer and that they were getting on with their lives. That they were normal, and looked as normal as possible... We had a lunch here one day and a new woman she was really quite shocked that I was seven years down the track. So I think it was really good for them to see someone.

Maya situates her work with breast cancer patients as a means of repaying the support she received during her own treatment. Meeting other women with experiences of breast cancer enabled Maya to position herself within a framework of 'normal' people – she was able to untangle her identity as a breast cancer sufferer as someone outside the norm and see that she was not alone. An important component of Maya's account is her emphasis on seeing women who looked 'normal'. One can assume this means seeing a woman whose appearance has been restored to what it was prior to surgery, with no visible signs of breast loss. Fulfilling this social obligation Maya is able to 'give back' something by looking normal herself.

Michelle, 63, is married and a grandmother.

> I just felt that I was alive and I wanted to give something back to the community, because that was important to me, and also I suppose in a way, it's a way of coping.

Like Maya, Michelle positions her contribution to the Bosom Buddies volunteer program as enabling her to 'give something back'. For Michelle simply being alive is reason enough to become involved, giving her survival a meaning and purpose. Volunteer work is a means of ordering the chaos of her breast cancer experience, enabling her to deal with her own grief and fear while helping someone else with theirs.

Patricia, 54, a public servant, divorced and a mother, attends the Cancer Council Breast Cancer Support Group regularly.

> When I was going through the chemo, which was a few months, I didn't feel all that wonderful and it was pretty scary and there were two other women going through it, one was a month ahead of me

and one was a month behind, and we supported each other quite well. And so that was really important. But it was good to see people, talk to people who were three and five years down the track. And know that, yes, you could survive. There were a couple of people who had lost all their hair from the chemo. And I didn't lose mine. That made me think I was pretty lucky. So there is a lot of that. But also I think the support, like if you do need to cry, the help of other women. But also the humour of the thing. It's a really good group. It's called black humour laughing about the situations and all that sort of stuff. And that was really positive for me. I guess now I don't have that need for the support because I actually think that I can give something back now. I like to think I can.

Patricia continues to attend the support sessions *for others*, her presence being a symbol of hope and survival. She views her role in the group as being one of support, feeling she no longer needs the support in return. Although she justifies her participation in this way it is hard to imagine she does not draw strength and comfort from the group. For Maya, Michelle and Patricia paying back the support they received is a necessary part of their continuing breast cancer experience. This new role gives significance to their continuing personal survival.

Patricia situates herself as lucky compared to other women because she did not lose her hair during chemotherapy. She suggests that another important function of the support group is being able to draw comparisons between her own and other women's experiences. In doing so Patricia is able to position herself amongst the social order of the group.

'*Only* a lumpectomy': Hierarchy in breast cancer support groups

While in hospital recovering from surgery and having daily radio-therapy treatments, Eileen, 47, was visited by a 'survivor' eager to offer her support and experience:

I guess everybody's experience is different. I think the woman who came to see me had possibly a worse time, she did actually have a breast removed and her attitude was sort of, well 'you *only* had a lump removed'. I felt like she'd been through much worse than I was going through so she probably needed more support than I needed...She also had lymphoedema, and all the bad things had actually happened to her. I guess we probably talked a bit more about her experience that mine. I guess I should just look at it that, yes, I am fortunate that I am on the lower rung.

Perhaps trying to make Eileen feel 'lucky', the woman from the support service only acts to alienate her. Within the framework created by this volunteer Eileen is situated at the lower end of the scale, denying her permission to fully participate in the 'breast cancer experience' as it is defined by the volunteer.

At one Cancer Council Breast Cancer Support Group meeting I attended one woman (Patricia) sobbed quietly as others spoke candidly about their mastectomy experiences. At the end of the session two women approached me, feeling they needed to explain her behaviour. I was informed that this was a regular occurrence, because 'you know, she's just had a lump removed'. When I spoke with Patricia later in an interview she described feeling that she did not belong or even have a right to be at the support group. Being unable to participate in discussions about loss of femininity and womanhood through mastectomy meant regardless of whether her own experience elicited these emotions she was cast outside the majority of the group. Grief and extent of surgery became a currency when women traded stories, situating women within a hierarchy of grief and loss. Anna, 50, has no hesitation articulating this hierarchy:

> There is a really funny serious story to be told in some of the support groups. Lowest pecking order is the lumpectomy, you know, you really can't consider yourself as really having cancer at all. You know, what would they know. And, um, the highest pecking order is the bilateral. And, um, there's a pecking order in between. It's really quite funny. Um, and of course the lumpectomy might have been quite as severe and invasive a cancer as ever the bilateral had. I had a bilat, so no worries, I was right up there.

To be 'right up there' is to have experienced the full extent of breast loss.

Whilst most feedback about support and advocacy groups is positive, not everyone credits these groups as wholly positive and supportive. As the accounts of Eileen, Patricia and Anna illustrate, the extent of surgery can impact on one's sense of belonging within a breast cancer community. In addition to physical characteristics, time, energy and the 'right' attitudes and belief systems also aid progress in one's breast cancer career.

The 'right' breast cancer identity

Rita spoke to me about her dealings with the BCAG Victoria:

> There has been a lot of unpleasantness in the group. I don't know if it's the natural history of community groups, but I think it's because there is a lot of people with a lot of anger and a lot of agendas with wanting to change things. The need to change things has I think got in the way of sensitivity to other peoples feelings, and other peoples desire to be included. And I sort of stopped being involved very much because it started to get very, very unpleasant. And I can see at a distance because of my involvement in community work why that need to do something with your anger, the need to change things is totally overwhelming and overpowering, and people sometimes behave insensitively because that's what they're trying to do. But it can be sad for the individuals who are then left out because the people with the most energy get to do what they want.

High emotion and differing personal agendas all affect the politics of advocacy groups. For an organization that is made up of women who have been or are ill, simply getting to the meetings can pose a challenge. Rita goes on to talk about how desperate she was to be involved with the group but was excluded from being part of various decision-making processes again and again because she could not be present. Rita told me that on a number of occasions she suggested to the committee that women unable to attend be emailed proceedings and given a chance to vote by mail on larger issues. According to Rita this idea was dismissed as too much of a hassle. In a community where a physical presence may be challenging it was a case of survival of the fittest. Several letters she wrote complaining about this and offering suggestions went unanswered. Rita suggests it is the stronger women with more 'energy' who tend to dominate such groups and are able to steer the direction of the organization to suit their own personal agendas.

The Australian supplement to Sharon Batt's (1994) *Patient No More* suggests that one can conclude that on the whole cancer charities in Australia are dominated by interests of various medical and pharmaceutical industries that control the treatment of and research into breast cancer (1994: 295). However, the BCAG notes that things are changing. For example, the appointments of consumer representatives on various cancer boards are applauded for putting the real issues for women on the agenda and demanding space for women's voices. While representatives are becoming increasingly visible, *how* these representatives are chosen and *who* they represent deserves critical attention.

Getting a 'seat at the table'

The 'Seat at the Table' project, run by the BCNA, is the main channel through which women with experiences of breast cancer become consumer representatives. The BCNA does the work to recruit consumers, sending out application forms in newsletters and constantly encouraging women to sign up. Women's details are entered into a database from which they can be chosen when their credentials are required. For example, if the NBCC needs someone for their Psychosocial Clinical Practice Guidelines steering committee, the BCNA committee (made up of BCNA members, state representatives and the national coordinator) determine what consumer attributes that position requires. These details are entered into the database and a list of suitable applicants produced. Nomination forms are then sent to these applicants who can decide if they are interested in the job and send in more details about themselves. The applicants are reviewed and considered by an 'undisclosed selection panel' (BCNA, 2003b) who ultimately decide who gets the position. Recommendation by committee members is one of the strongest ways to gain a 'seat at the table'. Personal relationships with committee members is therefore to the applicant's advantage.

Reviewing the list of consumer representatives on the BCNA website reveals that a core group of women sit on multiple boards simultaneously. The following woman's account raises complaints and comments I have heard consistently whilst carrying out my research.

I stayed in close contact with Jenny, 46, after our initial interview and she phoned with regular updates about how she was progressing in trying to get a 'seat at the table'. Diagnosed with breast cancer at 29 and again at 39, resulting in a bilateral mastectomy, Jenny thought she would be a great consumer representative. She had lived in rural NSW at the time of her second diagnosis and felt she could discuss the needs of both young women with breast cancer and women in rural areas. She completed the 'Science and Advocacy Training Programme' (a prerequisite for being a consumer representative) run by the NBCC. She lodged an application form and waited to be contacted. After the advocacy training she was incredibly excited and wrote what she describes as a 'wonderful submission' to represent country NSW women on the National Trials Panel in Darwin. She received no response and assumed she was not chosen. After a number of emails flaunting her credentials she was asked to make comments on papers via email; however, she never received anything to comment on.

When a survey from the BCNA arrived asking about issues that were important to women with breast cancer, Jenny dismissed the tick-a-box format choosing instead to respond in her own words. The head of BCNA responded to Jenny personally via email suggesting that with such a passion Jenny should perhaps sign up as a consumer representative. Assuming she was already included in the database, she made several attempts to contact the program coordinator, but her calls and emails were never returned. Reviewing the names of women who were consumer representatives she noticed that the same names kept coming up.

A few months later another questionnaire arrived, this time asking for women to volunteer for the 'Seat at the Table' project. Jenny admits that the comments she made on the form were critical of the project and instead of answering questions she used the survey to ask questions to the BCNA: How were consumer representatives chosen? Who chose them? Why did the same women appear on multiple committees and panels at the same time? There seemed to be no democratic voting process and women were never told what happened at the 'table' or if or how the woman representing her had made an impact. What did the consumer representative believe in? How would she know if they represented her beliefs?

Jenny's response was angry and honest and what she believed to be the thoughts of a number of women she had been talking to. Shortly after returning the questionnaire Jenny received a letter from the heads of the BCAG in Victoria and NSW. The letter described how upset they were by her response and stated that subsequently they did not think she would be a suitable representative on any forums. Seemingly blacklisted from the 'Seat at the Table' project and the advocacy groups involved with it Jenny found herself cast out of the breast cancer community. It seemed there was no room for criticism of the network or its functioning.

Jenny's supposed disloyalty to the breast cancer sisterhood extends further than her critique of the process of choosing consumer representatives. Where Jenny sees herself departing largely from the breast cancer community is in her refusal to wear prostheses. Jenny's belief that women should not be made to feel that they should wear prostheses was unwelcome at Bosom Buddies meetings and as a result she had to withdraw from her role on the committee. In our many discussions Jenny was concerned that she was an anomaly within breast cancer culture, and that perhaps she was just abnormal. Regarding the fashion parade she states:

They [the models] obviously enjoy the experience, but I think it's scary that, I think while people aren't prepared to publicly show that breast cancer is an injury to women and causes scarring and causes women to not have perfect bodies, until people are prepared to publicly show that, I don't think we'll ever advance breast cancer advocacy in the way that I think we need to. And I think the fashion parade perpetuates that 'put it in the closet and keep it covered up' ideology, because we don't want to offend anybody by showing ourselves with our boobless shape. And I think it's very sad.

The women who dominate support and advocacy groups seem to share the same attitudes and belief systems about women's mastectomized bodies. My interviews revealed that quite often women remain silent if they disagree. The space of the interview provided a setting where they could open up without offending the women who put so much time and energy into 'getting the message across'. There is nothing subtle in the message being given at the fashion parade. The post-surgical body is put on display with all its pretense, held up as a beacon of hope for women with breast cancer; they can still *look* normal after breast loss.

The challenge of 'going without'

> *But wait, there's more. Barbara commands our attention one last time as the President of Bosom Buddies, Sarah: Radical Mastectomy, Chemotherapy, Tamoxifen, Six Years Post-Diagnosis, walks up on stage. She presents a cheque to a representative from a research institute which tonight's fundraising will benefit. More applause. Then, as a special treat for the audience there is a door prize, care of one of the sponsors – One Thousand Dollars Worth of Cosmetic Surgery!*

The emphasis on appearance is poignantly portrayed in the cosmetic surgery door prize women are eligible for by attending the event. The post-surgical body is blatantly mobilized as something which is to be corrected. The event provides a public display of the restored body beautiful, a symbol of normalcy and femininity and successful 'life after breast cancer'. There is no shortage of positive appraisals for the Bosom Buddies fashion parade, with women in this study saying how wonderful and effective it is at promoting awareness. The consensus was that anything being done was better than nothing at all. However, what is revealed in the interviews is a message that is not privileged in breast cancer culture. Many women desperately seek permission to accept their body without having to 'cover up'. To show the mastectomized body truthfully would be granting permission to many women who remain covered up and silent.

Jenny was referred to a grief counsellor when she made her position publicly known at a breast cancer advocacy meeting. It was assumed that she had not come to terms with the reality of her post-surgical body and her positioning is pathologized as a psychosocial problem. On the contrary Jenny is confident with her body image and unashamed to publicly acknowledge that breast cancer is a disease that maims women's bodies. Rendering her attitudes 'unacceptable' and morbid illustrates the assumed norms within breast cancer culture.

One aspect of Jenny's account which stands out from other women's is her experience of the breast cancer volunteer who visited her in hospital:

> She came with a showbag, and she'd had a bilateral mastectomy, and that's why they got her to come to me. And she didn't wear anything. She had on just a jumper, and she said 'oh God, I never bother with all that, because why would you?', and I felt, phew. She was good, although the bag had the little fluffy things and stuff, which I went through and went 'oh my God'. But I never spoke to her again. She gave me her telephone number, and I think I've probably still got it, because it's like a security blanket or something. Not that I'm going to ring her. In a way it was nice to have her come, and nice to meet someone who'd had a bilateral mastectomy and was getting on with it.

The volunteer's open acceptance of her mastectomized torso was a relief for Jenny, and granted her permission to accept her post-surgical body without feeling pressure to 'cover up' with prosthetics. To Jenny, not restoring breast shape signals moving on with life and coming to terms with breast cancer and breast loss.

Having attended Bosom Buddies meetings where everyone gushed about the success of the fashion parade event, I used the private setting of the interview to explore further reactions. Women discussed experiences of being involved with the parade and also the possibility of women modeling without prostheses. For some women this was the first time they had articulated or thought about the possibility.

Maya, 53, talks about her experience of being in the fashion parade:

> I had been envious of women doing it for years. I'd been to most of the parades and thought, they are just so brave . . . they looked to be

having fun. That was one thing I decided, I would like to give it a go...I had my whole family and all my friends in the first couple of rows on one side and it was all such...you are alive and you are up there, the centre of attention. We look good, we felt good about ourselves. You know, if someone wants to get up there without [prosthesis], that would be fine. But I think that the aim of it has always been look how good we look, and look how much we can enjoy ourselves.

Maya is attracted to the fun and camaraderie the parade produces. The idea of a woman not modeling two breasted is situated as contradicting the aim of the event – to *look* good.

Christina, 57, a primary-school teacher, has had a lumpectomy and is awaiting news of whether she needs to have a mastectomy. She went along to the fashion parade for the first time, shortly after she had been diagnosed.

I thought it was wonderful. I was so full of admiration for those women, um, for daring to display their bodies, because they even wore lingerie. Um, for um, coming to terms with everything that had happened in their life, for being so positive, for making it, not confronting, but showing the world, whoever went to the fashion parade that we're still here, we're alive, life goes on, there's still plenty of things we do, we have many interests, you know. And that we're living proof that you can get through it, and come out the other side. And I like supporting things like that. But without a pros-thesis? I would have taken it totally in my stride, because we have disabled kids at work, and um, some are very disfigured, some of them behave in ways that are called weird, but you can sort of see past that to the person. So to me it wouldn't be as confronting as it would be to someone who's never been exposed to that sort of thing.

Christina likens women 'daring to display their bodies' to disfigured and disabled children she works with and frames the portrayal of the post-surgical body as potentially 'weird'. Christina suggests seeing women without prostheses could be very confronting to others.

Gemma, 33, featured in a fashion parade. I asked her how she would feel to see women modeling without restored breasts:

It would be really difficult for me. What they are looking at when they're seeing the women parade, is that they are not showing that they are wearing a prosthesis or they have had reconstruction, they are showing that they can be normal. If you showed a woman who had bilateral or had a mastectomy and went out there and modeled as is, they would be looked at differently, because they're different. And I don't know what response they would get. Hopefully it would be something really positive, because I think it would show a lot of courage to do that, or that's from my perspective anyway. I don't know whether I would be able to do that, um I probably would, just to show, yeah, this is what's happened, this is what is, this is what had to be done to overcome breast cancer. But yeah, interesting. I think it would be, it would probably be a good thing to do actually. Rather than, with women wearing prosthesis and modeling as they are they're showing that they're a whole woman, but underneath they're not . . . and maybe that story could be shown.

Gemma begins by expressing the difficulty she would have in dealing with women not wearing prosthesis. She is uneasy about the prospect as it contradicts the message of the evening – that women can be normal after breast cancer. However, as she talks she begins to think that maybe without prostheses a more positive message might be sent and decides she might consider it (Gemma had recently had her breast reconstructed so she actually could not model 'without'. She does not make this point though.) As she considers this further Gemma suggests that when wearing a prosthesis the models are displaying a pretence that 'underneath' they are not the 'whole woman' they appear to be. As Gemma's thoughts on the subject develop she highlights a tension between appearance and reality.

Similarly, Eileen suggests:

> I don't think it would be confronting. In fact I think it would probably be more honest and more accepting.

Petrea, 49, had a breast reconstruction and was the secretary of Bosom Buddies at the time of writing. On the subject of women modelling without prostheses she says:

> I think actually that it could be done and . . . I think that if someone has to wear a prosthesis I think that's all for . . . well I think it's often for the benefit of the rest of us, to make other people feel comfortable and not the woman herself. I think it would be very confrontational for some people if we did do it that way. And I have had debates but

so far that has never been considered. I know there is one woman I have noticed [Jenny], and she wrote in the newsletter once, did you see that? So I have been saying that sort of privately to a few people. But when she came out straight off and said it, and she is getting around with no prostheses and she teaches school. She just doesn't care. Accept her as a person. And she allowed me to express that. So I'd like to see more of it.

SC: And how do you think that could happen?

It has to be a decision that a woman herself makes. And then also you shouldn't be getting someone else saying, doesn't she look terrible because she doesn't wear a prosthesis. If we stopped being bitchy to one another it might help too.

Petrea feels she is unable to publicly discuss issues about not wearing prosthesis, suggesting the concealed mastectomy is a body 'for others'. Jenny's refusal to hide her mastectomized body gives Petrea permission to express her own concerns. Petrea feels her insights have come too late, now that she has had a reconstruction. Prior to meeting Jenny she felt unable to explore and express alternative feelings about the post-surgical body that lay outside dominant discourse. Petrea suggests that deciding not to wear a prosthesis is difficult, not being 'bitchy' to one another being an important factor in inhibiting this process. She alludes to a hierarchy that places alternative images of the post-surgical body as unacceptable.

Without prompting, Diane, 59, expresses that she would like to see models without prostheses:

Yes, I think it's [the fashion parade] terrific. I know it's probably an impossible thing for them to achieve, but it would be terrific to see someone up there who's not wearing a prosthesis, that's all. Someone game enough, or who David Jones would allow model the clothes, especially the women who have had two mastectomies, bilateral mastectomies, that would be just terrific to see someone up there not having to put a prosthesis in to replace their breasts. It's a lot harder to do when you only have one breast, I always wear a prosthesis, because I've got one side sticking up. Only a little bit [laughs], but still, it's flat on the other side [laughs].

SC: And why do you think it would be important for someone to get up there without wearing a prosthesis?

I think it gives a very positive message to women that they don't
have to have boobs to be people. I suppose I wear a prosthesis
because it keeps me balanced, but I just think you're just as much
balanced without either, and I don't think I'd wear prosthesis if I had
both breasts removed. And I think it gives a positive message that
you don't really need breasts to look good and feel good.

It is not just pressure from within the breast cancer community that
inhibits women's freedom to 'go without' at the fashion parade, but
also pressure from David Jones, the major fashion outlet who provide
the clothes for the event. In 1980 Audre Lorde drew attention to the
lack of clothing tailored to the mastectomized body (1980: 52) and
nearly 25 years later women must still conform to norms dictated by
clothing manufacturers, having to deny the reality of their body in the
process. Diane challenges dominant discourse by suggesting that breasts
do not complete or determine a woman's identity; that breasts do not
necessarily equate to *looking* or *feeling* good.

Barbara, 62, who organizes the fashion parade, spoke to me about her
concern that so many women have problems with their body image
after breast cancer surgery. Since she is a Bosom Buddies counsellor I
asked her how she helps women who come to her with issues to do
with body image:

Well, I tend to say your body, as far as I'm concerned, is the shell of
the person, and it's the person inside that counts. And because of the
prosthesis that they have nowadays, nobody can tell. And there's
one woman that I'm dealing with at the moment, and I'm going to
jolly well make sure she comes along to the fashion parade, because
if you see women up there in underwear and sleepwear, and they can
still just look as glamorous and sexy...looking at them as far as I
could tell they're a normal, everyday person.

Barbara emphasizes the aim of the parade is to *look* normal, not reveal
the truth about what lies underneath the prosthesis. The prosthesis is
described as enabling sexiness and glamour and normalcy. However, it
is also explicitly situated as a façade.

I asked Barbara how she would react if someone wanted to go in the
parade without a prosthesis.

If someone came to me now and said they wanted to, I would accept
them, but they would also need to be accepted by the fashion

boutiques, because if you're a person with just one breast, clothes are not going to hang as well. So this is something that you have to discuss with them before you would accept them, because, I don't see any problem with that, but the fashion houses may have a problem. It's something I've never actually brought up with them. And I think actually it's something I will bring up with David Jones now that you've mentioned it.

Although Barbara seems quite enthusiastic to me about the possibility of women not wearing a prosthesis, the next fashion parade is exactly the same as the last. It was never mentioned in discussions about the event at subsequent meetings I attended.

A dangerous discourse

Whilst it is important not to reduce breast cancer culture to something which is without diversity, despite differences which may exist the hegemonic need to restore normalcy through breast restoration is maintained. The ideals of mainstream 'pink advocacy' are located within a frame that situates the female body as something which is an object 'for others', and relies on stereotyped hyperfeminine images. Symbolized by varying pink hues, breast cancer culture reproduces soft, ladylike representations of women and their bodies with mastectomy situated as an invisible and unspeakable consequence of breast cancer.

Exemplified in *Pink Ribbon* magazine, breast cancer advocacy produces a discourse on women's mastectomized bodies using feminizing and infantilising tropes. This discourse constructs the post-surgical body as desexualized, ugly and abnormal and necessitating concealment at all times. It assumes a homogenous response to breast loss and fails to recognize that women are diverse and have diverse interests and needs. Instead breast cancer culture promotes an aesthetic hegemony tied to the norms of white, heterosexual, middle-class, commodified femininity. This is enacted in events like the fashion parade and discursively produced in texts aimed at women with breast cancer. These enable the mobilization of certain understandings and meanings that locate the mastectomized body as needing to be repaired and reconstructed in order to recover from a breast cancer crisis.

To aid that recovery are breast cancer volunteers who act as physical representations of the norms advocacy discourse produces. Presenting two-breasted and handing out 'fluffy ducks', these volunteers do more than simply 'give back' support they received, they simultaneously reproduce the post-surgical body as needing to be covered up and kept secret. The network of breast cancer advocates also provides a frame in which women can position themselves and others. Whilst breast amputation remains largely invisible in advocacy it acts as a currency with which women can be located hierarchically. In addition, individual breast cancer demographics translate into a new identity. A 'complete' breast cancer experience, including the full extent of breast surgery and treatment and then successful 'survival', can help one's breast cancer career. Women who have not shared the full experience are situated as unable to participate in discussions of loss of femininity or womanhood. A discussion of one woman's experience of trying to become a consumer representative illustrates how strongly women 'at the top' safeguard the ideals of breast cancer advocacy. Women who have differing views or understandings are excluded and silenced.

I have argued that while pink advocates would have us believe the overwhelming majority of women want and need to conceal their post-surgical body, in private discussions women openly and enthusiastically consider the possibility of not doing so. Using the fashion parade as an example, women in this study began to consider the use of prostheses as a pretence and that the restored body does not simply signal a 'complete' self. Instead the public display of the one or no breasted body at an event such as the fashion parade was situated as something which could be very positive, illustrating that women do not need breasts to look and feel good about themselves.

Individual and public challenges to the norms produced within breast cancer culture have the potential to grant other women permission to accept their post-surgical body. In addition a space would be created where the one or no breasted female body could be normalized, eliminating the expectation of women to 'cover up' and enabling women to explore for themselves what breast loss means. The aesthetic demands of society are presently unable to tolerate physical diversity or disability, and the breast cancer movement currently supports such limitations. Alternatively it could be helping promote acceptance for physical diversity.

4
Practices and Prostheses

Introduction

A woman stands, her naked back turned slightly away from the camera. Her head is cocked gently to one side, her age distinguished only by her cropped, bottle golden hair. A shadow over her face reveals only that her eyes are downcast. A beige satin nightgown drapes around her lower back and her hands gently cup her new 'Luxa Contact' prosthesis. Slightly darker in colour than her own complexion, the device sits closely to her skin with a natural drape and just a hint of nipple. The accompanying text reads:

> With the introduction of Luxa Contact, you can rest assured that it's finally here. The life-changing breast form you have been waiting for. A breast form that self-adheres, simply and directly to your body. Giving you total convenience. Natural comfort. Personal freedom. And that all-important 'it's part of me' sensation.[1]

Bordered in soft pink and mauve pastel, this advertising brochure describes one of many prosthetic devices currently available to the mastectomized woman. The world market for 'Breast Care' products, prostheses and post-mastectomy bras and swimwear, is estimated at $130 million and steadily increasing annually.[2] Manufacturers claim that women of all ages can find a prosthesis that approximates the 'shape and drape' of their existing breast, and they can be purchased in a variety of skin colour tones, with or without a nipple and areola. The internal composition of newer breast prostheses may consist of water, silicone, glycerin or latex, and the skin of the prosthesis is usually a lightweight, hypoallergenic plastic film of silicone.

This chapter examines the commodification of the post-surgical body by prosthesis companies, the medical profession and cancer organizations. All three provide powerful discourses that situate the post-surgical body as incomplete and abnormal in the absence of two breasts. Furthermore, to not restore the body to its pre-cancer appearance is to not fully participate in the recovery process. The mobilization of the prosthesis as a nexus between body and self is examined.

When in hospital recovering from breast surgery women are given an 'emergency' prosthesis made from cotton wool, commonly termed a 'fluffy duck'. Usually the woman's bra is whisked away at some point during her stay; tended to by an anonymous sewing lady, it arrives back, pouch affixed, ready to be filled. Once post-operative swelling has subsided, the newly mastectomized woman is ready to visit a qualified 'prosthesis fitter' who will measure her and work out the prosthesis that corresponds to her post-surgical body.

'Be free and be yourself again' is the slogan at Colleen's Post-Mastectomy Connection, the first shop of its kind to open in Canberra and one of only a few in Australia. The shop deals exclusively in post-mastectomy products: bras, bathers, prostheses and prostheses cases. Waist-high vases of artificial sunflowers fill the waiting room, testimony to Colleen's effort to make the shop unlike a sterile hospital environment. The fitting room is spacious, the walls lined with shoebox size cartons which hold the prostheses. There is a dressing table with a small mirror, big enough for a woman to see herself from waist up.

Women must make appointments and can bring along as many family or friends as they want. Colleen encourages women to visit her prior to their surgery to alleviate any anxiety they may have about becoming breastless. As prostheses cost from around Aus$200 to Aus$400 each, it is recommended women be fitted professionally. Colleen says this is essentially to get the 'mechanics' right and to get a prosthesis that will achieve the right 'drop' for each individual. An appointment may last for up to two hours as the woman tries on as many different prostheses as possible, searching for the one that she likes best and which most resembles her other natural breast. Clients are encouraged to jump up and down and lie on the floor in order to get a practical insight into how their new prosthesis will 'act' in different situations.

Women can choose products ranging from lightweight shoulder pad–like prostheses made from foam (that have the unfortunate tendency to creep from the bra and expose themselves at the most inappropriate times), to the high-tech silicone gel prostheses with an adhesive back which stick to the skin, ensuring ultimate discretion (see Figures 4.1a, b and c).

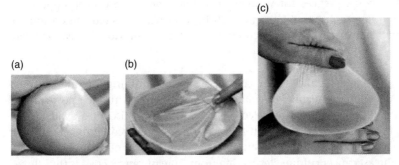

Figure 4.1 (a) The standard triangular shaped silicone breast form; (b) An adhesive-backed prosthesis; (c) A partial 'shell' breast form, recommended for women who have had a lumpectomy or reconstruction.
Source: Photos taken from http://www.coloplast.com/products, 2003a.

Women who want to wear a prosthesis, but for whom the cost or accessibility to a fitter is a consideration, have created their own prostheses out of materials available such as cloth stuffing, socks, rice and birdseed. Directions can be found on the Internet outlining how to make a breast prosthesis out of nylon stockings and millet.[3] However, women are warned that in warm humid climates, the organic materials may sprout.[4]

Iris Marion Young suggests that breasts are the most visible sign of a woman's femininity and the signal of her sexuality. She argues that

> However alienated male-dominated culture makes us from our bodies, however much it gives us instruments of self-hatred and oppression, still our bodies are ourselves. We move and act in this flesh and these sinews, and live our pleasures and pains in our bodies. (1990: 192)

Young argues that the integration of breasts with a woman's self is seriously denied in the events of a mastectomy. Instead breasts are considered to be detachable and dispensable.

Breast surgery, whether it is having a lump removed or bilateral mastectomy, is an assault on the body not only in a physical sense but also in a psychological sense. Kasper suggests that:

> in the process of managing a health crisis the women are also forced to renegotiate their sense of themselves as women. Indeed, the

consequences for women of losing a breast to cancer surgery are far-reaching and extend well beyond the expected dimensions of a health crisis to become a social and emotional crisis as well. (1995: 204)

Chapters 2 and 3 were concerned with examining the linguistic and social mechanisms women use to come to terms with their post-surgical bodies. Chapter 2 revealed a lack of positive discourse available for women to draw on when articulating the changed landscape of their bodies and Chapter 3 examined the reproduction of this silence within breast cancer culture. Recovering from a breast cancer crisis is thus linked with restoring breast shape and conforming to dominant notions of femininity. But these tropes which situate women's post-surgical bodies as incomplete and lacking femininity and sexuality are also materially produced. How is the post-surgical body materially defined and constituted?

The prosthesis is marketed as a device that aligns the post-surgical body with wellness and normalcy. Thus, the prosthesis is a point of convergence where self and body *appear* to be in harmony. What follows is an examination of the meanings women attribute to their mastectomy and the ways they successfully and unsuccessfully attempt to integrate the prosthesis into their self and daily life; how issues of body image are linked to femininity and identity in information booklets given to women during their illness; how these texts connect emotional and physical recovery to restoring breast shape; and finally, the powerful influence of prostheses manufacturers who link traditional notions of how the female body should look and act with recovery from a breast cancer crisis. Using themes of science and technology, liberation and femininity, and metaphors of being 'complete' and 'natural', advertisements for prostheses not only sell the usefulness of their devices but market certain understandings and meanings of the post-surgical body. Finally, by examining the daily practices of prostheses, discrepancies emerge as the prosthesis as a nexus between body and self is revealed to be unstable.

Meanings of mastectomy

One of the first questions asked in the interview was whether women were scared of losing their breasts when they were first diagnosed. Almost without exception the answer was 'no'. Fears were associated with dying, with the 'Big C' and with their chances of survival. Then there were fears associated with what chemotherapy was and how it would affect their body, and whether or not their hair would fall out.

It thus cannot be assumed that all women will make a connection between breast loss and femininity. Jenny, 46, is perplexed by this common association:

> If I had a husband where your whole sexuality was based on your boobs, and you weren't able to accept your sexuality, you know to feel that way without them, that would be pretty traumatic. I don't really know. To me, it just seemed strange to be a feminine thing, and people think that when they get them chopped off they don't have their femininity or something. Because I can't get my head around it, why it's such a big deal, I just don't get it. And I think it's better to have your life, and I cannot imagine hanging on to my boobs if that was a choice between life and death. Having boobs or dying, I mean, uh?

For most women the choice between life and a breast is not really a choice at all. Jenny talks about her mastectomy:

> Initially it's a shock, then you have all these tests, and you keep thinking well if it's spread they're not going to operate, then you think oh, if it's in my lung they won't operate, then you think if it's in there they won't operate, if it's here they won't operate, so when they say they're going to operate, it's like winning lotto, and you say GO! Go for it, whatever you want, chop it off. It's like a bonus at the end of this very long tunnel of trauma and pain.

In this instance the surgeon's decision to perform a mastectomy means relief for Jenny, it means that the cancer has not spread and that after the operation she will most likely be free of cancer. Jenny describes her breast surgery positively in the light of other cancer surgery people experience:

> At least boobs are like an extension of your body, so when they're chopped off it's really not affecting anything. To think that you have a brain tumour and have someone go in and take something out, it seems to me it would be a lot harder to get your head around. But chopping boobs off, it's not like taking a leg off, you can still walk around, you've got your mobility. And nobody sees the scars generally, and it's not that big an imposition really.

Gemma, 33, was diagnosed eight months ago:

> Between the lumpectomy and mastectomy I researched a lot, and read a lot about it, just to make sure that what I was being told was correct, and that I was being guided along the right path, and that he [the surgeon] wasn't just doing surgery for the sake of doing surgery, and that kind of thing. So by the time the surgery came around, I was quite calm and resolved to the fact that this was what needs to be done, let's get it over and done with, let's get the cancer out of my body, let me get back on with my life. I was more, I was upset after the lumpectomy, um, because I still had obviously a path to go through, and still at that stage we weren't sure whether the cancer had gone or not. And it hadn't, so I was really quite comfortable with the mastectomy at the end of the day, not comfortable, but resolved to the fact that this was what I needed to make me well.

Gemma's mastectomy means that the cancer is out of her body and she can get back on with her life. Although she is cautious in making sure it is not 'surgery for the sake of doing surgery' she sees it as a necessary trade-off to make her well again.

Lynette, 59, has been diagnosed with breast cancer twice, once nine years ago and again six years later. She describes her mastectomy:

> I was fortunate, they caught it in the early stages. That was a relief for me because at that stage I didn't have to go and have further treatment, radiation. I hadn't had a lumpectomy, I had a mastectomy. The reason why he [the surgeon] decided on that was because it was a certain type of cancer. And that's what they make the decision on. And I put my life in his hands because he was the expert. At no stage did I want a second opinion because I was satisfied that he was doing everything possible and I was satisfied in myself that I was making the right choices along the way. And that was really the only choice that I could make. I had nothing after that, no radiation, no chemotherapy, no tamoxifen.

Like Jenny, Lynette's mastectomy is a 'relief'. The operation means no further treatment and she is happy with the outcome. She describes her second diagnosis:

> I had six wonderful years of regular check ups, every year, every six months I would have a blood test, every year I would have another mammogram and just out of the blue, it was a yearly check up again.

I had no signs of any lumps again. But I had three tumours, had no relationship to the one in my left breast, and two different types. So really I had three different types of cancer in two breasts. The next step [it was] a bit of a shock first of all, but I could handle it so much better. I knew I wasn't going to die. We knew straight away, there was no lumpectomy or anything. It was just a natural progression. And that was one of the up sides, it evened me up. Because I did find that I was having posture problems.

Lynette situates her second mastectomy as inevitable. The routinized management of her body means that she had come to terms with the likelihood of recurrence and was thus prepared for the second diagnosis. The second mastectomy was a positive for Lynette as her body was physically realigned. She goes on to tell me her subsequent mastectomy enables her to wear two identical prostheses.

Jenny, Gemma and Lynette all frame their breast surgery as ultimately positive, as a relief, a trade-off, practical and akin to winning the lottery. Prior to surgery their breasts are dangerous and the mastectomy frees them of the immediate threat of cancer and death.

Lynette describes the first time she looked at her mastectomy site:

The first day I thought, oh well I am going to have to look at this. So I looked at it and I thought, oh that's not too bad. And I think it all depends on you as a person and how you feel your body image is. And I was not a size ten person that has always had a beautiful face. I have never been like that, never in my life. So there was nothing much for me to lose. So I have never been ashamed of me as a person and what I look like. I just dress accordingly.

Lynette makes reference to the connection of sense of self 'me as a person' and body image. Breasts are simultaneously constructed as superficial and an important locus of self. She alludes to having already come to grips with her sense of self as a woman with a large figure, dismissing issues of body image as therefore irrelevant to her.

June, 64, was diagnosed 12 months prior to the interview. She has had radiotherapy and was going through chemotherapy at the time of writing. She talks about seeing her mastectomy for the first time and what it meant having a breast removed:

That was the least of my worries. I just thought, this is coming out and that's all there was to it. And I knew what it would look like. I thought it looked worse than what actually [others] I'd seen. I worked at a hostel and I had seen a lady there which looked much better than what mine actually does. And I've seen Bill's [husband] mother, she had a mastectomy too. So I saw hers. And both those ladies had better mastectomies than I had. It was so nice and neat whereas mine... actually I think he's left mine so that I can have a reconstruction job done. So I think that's why, sort of leaving more there...When it was done it was pretty ugly. But I have come to terms...took a while to come to terms with that. Of losing it. Yes, you have lost something.

While June's mastectomy was the 'least of my worries', she is disgruntled by the cosmetic result. Although she never suggested she considered having a reconstruction, the surgeon leaves excess skin there just in case. She reflects that in losing her breast she has lost 'something' referring to a grief for more than simply physical loss.

Christina, 57, is awaiting results that will determine whether or not she will have a mastectomy. She talked to me about her feelings towards the possibility of losing her breast:

A breast is a small price to pay for a life, you know. And certainly I'm not a person who, um, focuses on the body that much, you know, so, and I also know that there are all these modern gadgets now.

The threat of breast loss is cushioned by the knowledge of 'modern gadgets' that are available – prostheses. While physical appearance is described as secondary to overcoming life threatening disease, historical, social and cultural meanings ascribed to breasts prefigure the difficulties women will face when breast loss occurs.[5] Anticipating the challenge surgery may have to her body image, sense of femininity and public appearance, Christina buys a prosthesis, just in case:

I bought a prosthesis quite comfortably, and not just for the vanity, but just because it makes sense to normalize yourself. I don't like to be caught in my grubbiest clothes when I've come out of the garden all sweaty, I'm vain enough for that. But I would wear one, for the balance, you know. Because I don't think you need to shout to the world, look I'm weird, because it's confronting to other people.

For Christina, the prosthesis is an opportunity to normalize herself, her purchase being a pragmatic one. Just as breasts are situated as dispensable in the threat of cancer, they are replaceable with the availability of prostheses.

Treatment for cancer and breast loss alters a woman's physical appearance. Hair loss and skin pigment changes can result and women may seek to recover the body through various cosmetic treatments such as wigs, make-up and vitamin supplements. Whilst these changes require 'body work' for relatively short periods of time, mastectomy can require more constant renegotiation. Jenny describes the 'reality' of her mastectomized torso:

> The one thing that is bad about not having boobs, is that your stomach pokes out. So you become this pear shaped person, and I think that as you get older your stomach gets bigger, and I think if you had boobs it would not be as obvious.

Although Jenny is concerned about the weight she has gained since her surgery, she has no intention of having breast shape restored:

> Because I can't see the point. I can't see the point of having it so that your clothes hang better, I mean, or so that you have this lumpy front. If that's all you've got to worry about, it's nothing, you're still alive, I mean, I just couldn't be bothered. One of my girlfriends reckons she's worked out at the gym for years to try and get a chest looking like mine [laugh].

For some women, breasts are constituted as purely physical attributes that complete a woman's status as woman and as 'normal'. While Jenny is able to maintain a positive outlook because she is 'still alive' after breast cancer, for others this quickly fades as they are faced with strong social discourses that frame their post-surgical body as unacceptable. Prostheses are offered as a façade to project status as woman, and furthermore as recovered.

Integrating a prosthesis into the self

The link between 'wellness' and normalcy is integral to making the post-surgical body in breast cancer. Not only is the reestablishment of a sense of wellness important, but 'looking' well is very important. In *looking* well and normal a woman presents herself as 'recovered'. Thus securing a return to normality requires the successful presenting, monitoring and interpreting of bodies[6] so that no one may discover the 'truth' about a breast amputation.

Diane, 59, explains her need to get a prosthesis:

> I just wore a bra as soon as possible with a bit of stuffing in it, and as soon as I could I had a prosthesis. I was very, very keen to get the prosthesis, in fact I was too, I really acted too quickly, because I had too much swelling...I was rushing into trying to feel normal again, but that was all I wanted...I was just a pretty smart dresser, and it was a time in my life I felt quite physically good, and I just wanted to get that appearance back again, to go with all my clothes.

Diane's impatience to buy a prosthesis and 'feel normal again' positions the device as more than simply a precursor to recovery. Instead normalcy and wellness are depicted as being contingent upon regaining her two-breasted appearance.

For Anna, 50, the prosthesis is integrated totally into the self:

> I wore it 24 hours a day, never without it. It made me feel whole... I was never without it for a second. I didn't sleep with it on, uh, I had it beside my bed, and I put it on like you do your watch first thing of a morning, and I was never without it...going out, it was like brushing your hair, like, you just had to have it on.

Incorporating the prosthesis into her daily routine enables Anna to feel 'whole'. This metaphor for recovery suggests that without restoring her two-breasted appearance she is missing a part of her self. This 'whole' self is contained within an outward projection of normalcy. The intersection of normalcy, wellness and prostheses is done both by women who wear the devices and by the people and literature that market them.

The 'Breast Care Package'

A growing collection of research identifies the importance of access to information on women's decision making and self-esteem throughout their illness, and analyses have been done showing the importance of access to medical information.[7] Text-based literature is an important component of the information women receive during their illness. Written in lay terms aimed specifically at consumers, patients can take it home and read it at their leisure. This contrasts to the confusing medical terminology and varying opinions women may be receiving from oncologists, surgeons, general practitioners, counsellors and breast care nurses. Short, easily digested booklets are therefore a very powerful medium through which women access information and options.

In Australia, most women are offered a 'showbag' of information and post-mastectomy product brochures at some time during consultations or treatment. Compiled by hospitals and breast cancer organizations, this bag contains contacts for support groups and cancer societies. Included are booklets on adjuvant breast cancer therapy (radiotherapy, chemotherapy and hormone therapy), emotional and psychological issues and options for women before and after their mastectomy.[8] In addition the package contains two cotton wool 'emergency' prostheses.

Much of the information in these booklets relies on the premise that part of recovery is 'regaining your normal figure'.[9] From the outset, restoring the post-surgical body to its state prior to illness is linked to regaining 'wellness'. To refuse to wear a prosthesis is thus to not participate fully in the recovery process.

Implicit in discussions of restoring appearance is the idea that breast cancer challenges a woman's body image, sexuality and self concept. In consumer literature issues of body image and sexuality are dealt with cursorily and as matters of fact, and always in the context of relationships. One booklet offers this advice:

> Some women will find it difficult to adjust to the appearance of their body after their breast cancer treatment. Other women adjust quickly and with ease. You may feel physically unattractive. You may be worried about your partner seeing your body. You may wonder if and how sex will be affected. Some women feel sexually unattractive during and after treatment and avoid physical contact with their partner. Other women just don't feel like having sex for a while. Ask for affection when you need it. It is possible that your partner will be afraid of being insensitive towards you and so it may be up to you to let your partner know if you are interested in sex or other forms of affection such as cuddling or kissing. Talk about your fears and worries with your partner.[10]

Although body image and sexuality are acknowledged, no reassurances are made of the normality of the mastectomized body. No suggestions are offered as to how a woman may 'adjust' to this changed body, instead she is given a list of acceptable emotional responses and urged to negotiate her post-surgical body in terms of her own and her partner's sexual desire.

Emotions and Cancer includes discussion of body image explicitly within the context of advice for a woman's partner:

> Despite physical changes, your partner needs to know that you still love them and find them attractive. Try to see past your partner's physical appearance. Remind yourself of their other qualities that you find attractive: sense of humour, intelligence or personality... Touching or stroking the scar may help show your partner that you have accepted these body changes.[11]

Whilst this booklet urges partners to accept the mastectomized body through touching, no such encouragement is given to the woman herself to accept her altered corporeality. Similarly in a 'Breast Care Package' given to women at a hospital in Canberra, issues of body image are directed entirely at the partner:

> The woman who has undergone breast surgery has a number of sexuality issues to contend with. Firstly she has to come to terms with the changes to her body and body image. For some women, they can feel that their femininity has been challenged and coping with this change can take time. Secondly, she can be fearful of your reaction to seeing the scar/mastectomy or of you finding her unattractive and rejecting her as a sexual person and partner. It is a time when women feel particularly vulnerable. She may feel less desirable. Reassuring her of your love can assist your partner through this period.[12]

Located in third person, the mastectomized woman is situated as a passive recipient of the information, dependent on her partner's acceptance of her changed body. The text makes assumptions about how a woman defines her femininity, in this case as something located inherently within her breasts. How does one 'come to terms' with body changes? What mechanisms to 'cope' are available? Indications are given in the following 15 pages of the booklet which are dedicated to prostheses: where to buy them, how much they cost, where to find qualified prosthetic fitters, details of private health fund benefits and information about Prosthesis Schemes, where small amounts of government funding are available towards the cost of a first prosthesis. A pattern and instructions for a Bra insert in which the 'equipment' will sit are also included.

One can only conclude that overcoming emotional and sexual difficulties created by breast surgery is largely contingent on a woman's willingness to wear a prosthesis. What is important in these texts is not so much what is written, but what is not. No effort is made to grant permission to women to touch and accept their post-surgical body. Instead, prostheses are promoted both as being essential to restoring appearance and as a vehicle of normalcy.

Marketing prostheses

How a Breast Form is Born
A film by the Amoena-Coloplast Corporation (1992)

Soft instrumental music accompanies a montage of images:

A mother reading a story to a young child. An elderly couple ride bikes through a park, laughing. A middle-aged woman buys a shirt. An elderly couple stroll through the park and kiss. Another elderly couple laugh over a coffee in a café. A large family share a meal, all laughing. A middle aged couple fish, laughing.

The sweet, softly spoken voice of an American woman accompanies the images:

'At Amoena we have just one goal, to help women everywhere enjoy more fuller, active lives after breast surgery. Since 1975 our only business has been the design and manufacture of the most advanced post breast surgery products available . . .'

The viewer is taken to the factory floor: a man takes a breast form out of a machine, weighs it and places it on a large pile of other prostheses. Small steel devices glide across larger ones, men and women in white coats tend to different sized machines, turning knobs, adjusting gauges, mixing liquid in beakers.

'We take the time to fully understand the needs of our customers. That includes closely monitoring changing surgical techniques, testing each new design and refining it until it's as perfect as we can make it . . .'

Now to the offices. A man and woman sit in front of a computer examining a 3D prosthesis model. A 'designer' works at an easel, another moves different fabrics over a breast form.

'In terms of comfort, shape and natural feel, this process can take as long as five years to complete. When a new design is ready to join the Amoena family of products it is carefully produced using a combination of the most advanced technology and precision instruments and the concerned well

trained eyes and hands of our expert manufacturing team. Let us show you exactly how a breast form is born...'.

A series of images of men and women in white coats and gloves tending to different stages of the process are shown. The 'envelope' is sent to the 'pumping station' where is filled with 'filtered' silicone at a 'carefully monitored ratio'. The form is then sent to the oven. When the prosthesis 'emerges' it is 'thoroughly inspected for appearance, softness and colour'. This involves a man in a white coat standing in front of a pile of prostheses, picking up each one and squeezing and stroking them. Finally, the form is 'thoroughly cleaned' and given a matt finish to give it a 'soft, skin like feel'.

The voiceover offers a concluding monologue which accompanies images of women jogging, playing tennis and even an executive looking woman working at a desk:

'Along with comfortable, feminine post-mastectomy bras, the Amoena line of breast forms provides the softest possible alternative for women who have undergone breast surgery... We are dedicated to providing our customers with the finest handcrafted product and we never forget that a woman's confidence cannot be mass produced... And that what our customer is buying is not just a new breast form but a new beginning. Everything we do at Amoena is dedicated to making that beginning as beautiful as it can be'.

The marketing of prostheses not only sells the functionality of a tool but also produces certain understandings of the post-surgical body. Advertisements for prostheses produce notions of femininity, beliefs about how the post-surgical body should be presented and performed, and assurances of what the devices will enable women to do. These advertisements are thus useful in analysing the production of knowledge about the mastectomized body as it is framed as incomplete, abnormal and unhealthy. Furthermore, breast amputation is constructed as temporary, to be 'fixed' as soon as possible.

Promotional films, like the one described above, are available from manufacturers and sales representatives and are shown to support groups, LGFB workshops, and on request to professional prosthesis fitters. The juxtaposition of the sterile, machine-filled factory floor with the softly spoken feminine voice-over whispering about *Amoena*'s 'natural', 'hand-crafted', 'beautiful' products brings attention to the work that goes into transforming this inanimate object into something that can be integrated into a woman's sense of self. Above all, the message of the film, driven home by montage after montage of 'happy' women, is that wearing a prosthesis makes life better; and not just better than prior to wearing the device, but better than life was ever before. Indeed, *Amoena* offers a 'new beginning' promising a life more 'confident' and more 'beautiful'.

Framing the post-surgical body

In the sample bag from one Canberra hospital, advertisements from two major breast prosthesis manufacturers are included – '*Anita – Care*', a German manufacturer, and '*Amoena*', based in North America.

'*Anita – Care*' sells throughout Europe and Australia. The youthful models featured in its brochures pose against pastel backdrops, smiling and laughing. The women look unlikely to be masking the 'imperfections' their product aims to hide. On the front of the brochure the company's philosophy is outlined:

> A grain of sand becomes a pearl. A pearl is one of nature's ways of correcting an imperfection which has always fascinated mankind. Its perfect form, its delicate shimmer and wonderful method of creation makes it an exquisite adornment. Our breast prostheses were designed to provide a gentle and aesthetic option for women to correct an imperfection after breast surgery. Restoration of a feminine outline and comfort which is kind to the skin provide the basis for a new quality of life. Many breast prostheses are not made with this principle in mind as they have degenerated to purely technical products. For many women they therefore remain nothing more than a foreign body. Our careful product development and recollection of classical values as well as the true needs of these women and their sensitive emotional and physical situation are more important than ever before. In keeping with this philosophy, ahead of all competition, Anita® has independently created a pioneering holistic concept for breast prostheses, bras and swimwear.[13]

The '*Anita – Care* philosophy' presents the 'imperfect' post-surgical body as transient and the prosthesis as transforming a woman's mastectomized torso into an 'exquisite adornment'. An explicit link is made between their product's life-changing potential and the importance of restoring a feminine appearance. They claim that this connection is integral to their product's success, contrasting it with their competitors' negligence in allowing the prosthesis to be something that can never be integrated with a woman's sense of self.

Given that breast prostheses have similar compositions no matter which company manufactures them, one may consider how *Anita* can differ so much. However, they reveal their secret weapon is their 'recollection of classical values' and their sensitivity to women's emotional and physical situation. For the prosthesis to become more than a 'foreign body' there needs to be a fusion of material and subject that is both in the mind and on the chest. These 'classical values' are never detailed, but allude to notions of heteronormative femininity. Indeed, *Anita*'s 'holistic concept' is one that integrates the need for a restoration of *looking* and *feeling* feminine and normal. The prosthesis-clad body is in its truest sense a cyborg: a fusion of subject and material.[14]

Anita's philosophy brings attention to three dominant themes in prosthesis advertising: (1) claims to scientific and technological authority; (2) restitution of femininity and liberation to a new and better quality of life; and (3) metaphors of being 'complete', 'whole' and 'natural'. All three produce and perform particular understandings of the post-surgical body and at times emerge simultaneously, contradicting and overlapping one another.

Comfort, confidence and security

Amoena (manufactured by the Coloplast Corporation) is a self-proclaimed global leader in 'advanced medical adhesive technology'. Coloplast focuses on chronic care needs, which include wound care, appliances for ostomates and incontinent individuals, and products for women after breast surgery. According to their website, '*Amoena* is Latin for the beautiful, the lovely'.[15] They claim to be the world's leading brand of external breast forms and post-mastectomy bras. Unlike the *Anita – Care* brochures, the models featured in *Amoena* advertisements are breast cancer survivors, as stated on the back of each pamphlet, and their brochures are given authority by many anonymous testimonials.

The product brochure included in one information package details the *Amoena* range:

> As the world's leading brand of post-mastectomy products, Amoena is the choice of women who enjoy full, active lives after breast surgery. Amoena products allow you to pursue the lifestyle you choose with confidence, security and comfort. Amoena breast forms are available in many styles and shapes and sizes. All are individually handcrafted with a unique silicone mixture that gives a look and feel that's soft and natural. Whatever your body type, breast shape or type of surgery, there is an Amoena breast form to fit you ... Women of all

ages are discovering there are many ways to restore their appearance and renew their self-confidence following breast surgery.[16]

The 'individually handcrafted...unique silicone mix' secures the oxymoronic image that the prosthesis is both technical and individual, more than a generic device. Successful emotional and physical recovery is described as being dependent on returning the mastectomized body to its former self. The prosthesis *enables* women to be confident, secure and comfortable. They can be confident that no one will know the truth about their post-surgical body and secure that the prosthesis will not reveal itself. The restoration of appearance is aligned with a renewal of self-confidence enabling 'fuller active lives'.

The *Anita – Care* range includes 'comfort' prostheses which are light-weight and simple in design (a basic round shape without nipples) for use when swimming and over uneven scar tissue. Anita also offers breast prostheses for 'individual customization', which have variable volumes, ensuring 'perfect compensation irrespective of the post-operative effects, type of figure and the selected bra style'.[17] Their top buy however is the 'full prostheses with Flex-gap® system':

> This patented style has a special backing design (indentation) and a soft and natural silicone gel composition...The Flex-gap® system offers you the following advantages: close fit and softness, natural underbust shape, optimum cup shaping, natural movement; flattens when wearer is lying down.[18]

Like *Amoena*'s range, the above 'system' makes a claim to scientific authority through appealing to the technical wonders of the product whilst simultaneously being promoted as wholly 'natural'. This emphasis on the controlled technology of their product ensures a level of safety where women can be assured the prosthesis will not escape from the bra and reveal itself. The wearer can be sure she is safe from others knowing the truth about her breast amputation.

The *Amoena* brochure, 'What every woman who has had breast cancer should know: A guide to restoring your appearance, self-image and confidence'[19], outlines post-operative choices. These include breast prostheses, breast reconstruction or partial breast forms (shapers) for women who have had breast conserving surgery. *Amoena* also offers 'comfort during recovery' by way of a soft bra and 'fiberfill breast form' that is apparently less restrictive during the healing process. This is presented as being 'ideal for future activities such as gardening and flying'.[20] In addition, *Amoena* has a variety of breast form types with varying functions. For example, shapes include triangular, asymmetric and teardrop, and the prosthesis can be non-adhesive or attachable. Non-adhesive breast forms must be worn with a bra whereas attachable breast forms can be worn braless.

In one brochure for attachable prostheses the testimonial reads:

> My attachable breast form allows me to wear low cut dresses, swimsuits, feminine lingerie and designer bras. The best part is, I look wonderful![21]

Apart from making the wearer 'look wonderful' the attachable prosthesis enables freedom and femininity. But they go further:

> When you start wearing your new external breast form, you will experience a more balanced self – both physically from the weight of the form, and emotionally by a return of self-confidence.[22]

Although research indicates that no physiologic changes are experienced by women who wear under-weighted breast forms,[23] *Amoena* suggests that 'because the breast form's weight is supported by the chest wall, these breast forms help eliminate strain on the shoulders and back'.[24] In this statement the prosthesis is described as an accessory to be worn that enables both physical and emotional stability. In addition they claim that the form moves with the body:

> [A]llowing you full freedom of movement and complete confidence to pursue activities like tennis, golf, jogging and swimming.[25]

Although the advertisement at the beginning of the chapter describes the 'it's part of me sensation', this illusion is revealed as temporary when emphasis is placed on the importance of regular cleaning of the breast form:

> During the day, perspiration, powder, perfume, clothing and dead skin cells can build up on your breast form. If the breast form is not cleaned, eventually this build up may start to breakdown the exterior of the breast form and cause it to deteriorate early. Washing your breast form is easy. It can be done in the shower with you each day or in a basin.[26]

Having established that the prosthesis can be integrated totally into the self, the image of it deteriorating early and the breakdown of its exterior is a threat to bodily integrity. Getting the mechanics of the device working properly can further distance the wearer from the product:

> Amoena has created two beautiful bras – one underwire, one soft cup – that work as perfect partners with Luxa Contact. The unique two-layer design features a flowable gel back that contours to your body and gives you a close hug. It's best not to attach Luxa Contact when you think you might perspire more than normal. Instead, wear it with a CoolPad, inside the pocket of a post mastectomy bra. The key to wearing Luxa Contact with ongoing success is cleaning it thoroughly after each wearing, and Luxa Contact comes with a storage cradle, protective back covering, two CoolPads, marking pencil and an accessory kit that includes a cleaning brush, Amoena Breast Form Wash and an instruction booklet.[27]

Instead of becoming a part of the wearer, this excerpt describes the device more like a high maintenance friend, able to give a 'close hug'. Whether marketed as being a technical wonder or agent of security, freedom and femininity, prostheses are represented as integral to restoring physical and emotional health and well-being. In addition, prostheses are constructed as vehicles of normalcy and necessary if one is to be accepted back into a two-breasted society. As *Amoena* articulates so succinctly in the statement of its 'core purpose':

> To offer those individuals that have suffered a disabling condition, which may result in extreme embarrassment and discomfort, the opportunity to re-enter the community with a feeling of confidence and normality, where they will look and appear no different to those around them.[28]

Both prosthesis companies, *Anita – Care* and *Amoena*, work hard to establish that their products are more than simply technical. Instead they are promoted as being 'a part of you'. Women are encouraged to embody the device, become a cyborg. The prosthesis is given agency enabling femininity, normality, freedom, confidence, renewed self-esteem, full active lifestyle, balanced self, and improved quality of life. In this way these advertisements depict the post-surgical body as incomplete in the absence of breast restoration.

Breast prostheses are a multimillion dollar industry and marketing of these devices is embedded in a history of particular meanings and understandings of women and their bodies. While prostheses are supposed to become a part of the self and the body, this requires all kinds of material-specific practices. The post-surgical body is hidden and has to be kept hidden at all times, even while swimming or, as one brochure suggests, during a 24-hour flight. It is simultaneously being constructed as disfigured and as requiring concealment.

Prosthesis manufacturers work hard to mobilize the prosthesis as an all encompassing beacon of normality that will transform a woman's body to one that is socially acceptable. When examining the daily practices of the post-surgical body the stability of the prosthesis as enabling normalcy comes into question. A shift occurs when a woman's life begins to resemble that which was prior to illness and the prosthesis is no longer seen as an agent of freedom and confidence, rather the opposite as restrictive and problematic.

Getting 'back to normal'

For some women the full impact of losing a breast does not come until they have gotten over the 'surviving bit', when life is returning to normal, when they are going back to work full time or feeling well again after months of chemotherapy.

Anna, 50, suggests that

> When you have breast cancer all you think of is survival, so that takes you through the first few months, through your treatment, through your chemo, all that sort of thing. You don't really start thinking of the damaged woman bit until after it's all finished.

Thoughts about how breast cancer has more deeply affected her sense of self occur after treatment has ceased. Anna refers to these feelings – the 'damaged woman bit' – as a prefigured set of thoughts and feelings towards a corporeally challenged femininity, sexuality and identity. In being 'damaged' she situates herself as less than other women who have two breasts and less than the self she knew prior to illness. She is damaged both physically and emotionally.

Similarly, Sarah, 49, feels emotionally and physically isolated:

> I didn't really think at the time how I would feel later on, about the loss of the breast. When you're in hospital, and when you're still going through the shock of being told you've got cancer, you're in another world really. The real world doesn't come back to you until you start to recover really, and then get back to normal and that's

when you start feeling quite, you know…I'd be sitting in groups of women and I'd think, I'm different, and I look and feel different. But that came two and a half years later.

Sarah's return to the 'real world' signals to her how different she is since breast cancer and surgery. She is unable to regain status as 'normal' and is left emotionally and physically isolated. She is caught in two worlds belonging to neither the sick nor the well. She positions herself unlike other women with breast cancer and unlike women who have not had it.

Marie, 52, describes her feelings after the mastectomy:

> I'd been focusing on getting better, and it hadn't spread, and well, I was focusing on getting over the chemotherapy, recovering from that, and getting my hair back. And then when everything was back to normal, that was when it really hit me, and it hit quite hard…I just started getting depressed and [starting to cry] and I don't know, I guess I was getting a bit angry, really. Not realizing at the time, but a lot of the unresolved anger internally, and feelings of not being a complete woman.

For Marie, getting 'back to normal' has a different point of reference to that of Sarah. Marie is able to regain a sense of normality in her life but is unable to control internal feelings which surface as depression. Like Sarah and Anna, Marie's feelings of not being 'complete' signal a distancing of body and self and 'harmony' between appearance and reality begins to unravel.

Mathieson and Stam (1995) argue that it is the cumulative effect of the changes which result from diagnosis and treatment that lead to the woman's awareness that she has been transformed permanently by having cancer. These women spoke of feeling unprepared for feelings of grief and loss, of looking and *feeling* different. As women are expected to 'get back to normal' with no visible mark of their loss, society gives no permission to grieve for the amputated breast and provides no space in which such feelings can be dealt with.

Daily practices of prostheses

When status as 'normal' has been reached through using prosthetic devices problems can occur. As Jacqui describes,

> Prostheses aren't comfortable to wear. To wear them you always have to wear a bra. And I've always found it hard to get a bra to fit because

of the fact that I am wide and all that sort of stuff. And you don't have the same movement wearing a prosthesis. It's funny, I go to the gym without a bra on because I'm more comfortable. When you are moving your breasts move but your prosthesis doesn't. So when you are pumping iron it sort of creeps up out of your bra. It's much easier to move without one on.

During the hot weather, very hot, you have got this bit of plastic sitting against your chest wall, and if you sweat like I do... And they are very hot and I get a lot of rashes. So it would probably be more comfortable to have reconstructive surgery. Like in the long run. On a day to day basis. I would probably feel renewed.

Jacqui describes her prosthesis as a foreign object and something which causes her a great deal of discomfort. Discussions of the hassles of prostheses always lead to a discussion of the possibility of reconstruction as an alternative.

Stephanie, 53, also describes her prosthesis as entirely distinct from her body. She contrasts prostheses and reconstruction:

I think it's a pain in the neck. It's like to me breastfeeding or bottle feeding a baby. It's a strange analogy I suppose, because we're talking about breasts, that's not what I meant. You've got the equipment, you use it. Why would you go boiling up milk and doing all these false things, putting false foods into a baby, when you've got something natural to give them? So if I can be natural again, that's the way nature intended me to be..., you've got this thing you've got to clean it and sterilize it, and I've got this prosthesis I've always got to care for this and wash it, and what about the day when you don't get it washed. I mean there was one day when I washed the damn thing and it wasn't dry enough for me to wear it to work. And I'm thinking what the hell am I going to do? I can't go to work! No way was I going without it, you know?

To Stephanie, the prosthesis symbolizes something which is 'false' when there is a 'natural' alternative – a reconstruction. The extent of constraint she experiences when her prosthesis is temporarily unavailable convinces her of the positives of reconstruction.

Anna, 50, explains that one reason she sought reconstruction was to deal with the difficulties with sport:

I'd bend down to take a low ball at squash or something and if I'm not lucky it would come out... And my cancer was quite high up and I was left with a dent quite high up in my chest, about there [points to about 10cms below collar bone], and so even with special breast cancer swimmers it would come out, I really needed some like [pulls her top up to cover scar], and so I stopped swimming.

The prosthesis, rather than her post-surgical body, prevents her from playing sport. For Jacqui, Stephanie and Anna, wearing a prosthesis is severely restrictive. It inhibits movement when going to the gym or playing sport and requires high maintenance to remain wearable.

The confidence Sarah experiences when she first wears her prosthesis quickly diminishes as she is confronted with the daily practices of tending to it:

Well at first I liked it, because it felt like I had some breast, but before that there was nothing, there was one flat side – I wasn't back at work at that stage. I got the prosthesis quite early after I'd had the operation, and I had this newfound confidence all of a sudden, but then that just disappeared. I had to put this thing in, then I 'd end up pinning it in, to the bra, and it would fall out at embarrassing times, you know, and I felt that I couldn't, um, some of the clothing that I wore was a bit low, if I lent forward, the prosthesis would fall forward, and you could actually see between, you know [the prosthesis and chest wall], and that was a bit, you know. So, I had to have a reconstruction.

The language Sarah uses implies a lack of choice as the daily hassles of the prosthesis – pinning it, keeping a close watch so it does not fall out – means that she 'had to have' a reconstruction. She goes on:

At first I thought that I probably wouldn't have a reconstruction, because the prosthesis was there, and [unclear], and that was fine, but later on I realized there were heaps of problems involved in it, and not being able to – sometimes I'd be around the house with a t-shirt and no bra, and then someone would come to the door and I'd have to rush and put it all on.

The stress of possibly being caught without her prosthesis is further reason for Sarah to seek reconstruction as an alternative solution.

Petrea, 49, is defiant about not wearing a prosthesis 'for others':

I went in and got a prosthesis and I wore it once and I hated it. And I never wore it again. And so I went around for a whole year afterwards just flat on one side. And I got to the stage . . . I'd see people staring at me sometimes and I didn't really care very much . . . It just didn't feel like it was a part of me and I just didn't see the point of it. I thought, if I had my arm cut off, if it was going to be a useful thing, okay, but if it was just so other people wouldn't be horrified then it didn't seem any point to me. And yet on the other hand I went and then had a reconstruction.

Petrea cannot integrate the prosthesis into her self and subsequently can not see the usefulness of it. She is very articulate about her contradictory feelings, and the complexity and multiplicity of the experience is revealed as she goes on to get a reconstruction.

Gemma, 33, describes why she is looking into reconstruction:

Just to be normal. Just to feel that, um, yeah, I don't think I'd be comfortable with wearing prostheses for the rest of my life, I think I'd want to have a look at other surgical options, to just have reasonably normal tissue there, rather than having things that you stick on and take off.

In these women's accounts there are only two options in order to regain a sense of normalcy following mastectomy – to wear a prosthesis or have a reconstruction. Gemma is unable to conceptualize a return to normality using 'things' which she must 'stick on and take off'. A discrepancy emerges between breast restoration as a step in the recovery process and the experience of these devices. Far from being the agents of freedom, femininity and normalcy that manufacturers promote, women who wear the devices situate them as foreign objects which signal a distancing of their body and self. As a 'bit of plastic', these devices cause rashes and discomfort, require cleaning and drying and demand constant surveillance to ensure they do not reveal themselves or the truth about a woman's maimed body. These daily practices constantly reproduce the post-surgical body as damaged and incomplete and act only to emphasize how different these women's lives are since their breast surgery.

Conclusion

This chapter has outlined the ways the post-surgical body is discursively produced by prosthesis manufacturers and cancer organizations and how it is performed in everyday practices. I have argued that the meanings women attribute to breast loss are initially positive as mastectomy is situated as a trade-off for life. Knowledge of the availability of prostheses cushions the impact of breast loss, and prosthesis is understood as a mechanism to normalize the body and self. This knowledge is gained through the consumer-based literature women are given at the time of diagnosis and further emphasized in advertising brochures from prosthesis companies.

I have argued that the information women receive from organizations like the Australian Cancer Society contains the premise that part of recovery is regaining a 'normal' figure. From the outset restoring the post-surgical body to its state prior to illness is linked to regaining 'wellness'. In consumer literature the mastectomized woman is situated as a passive recipient of the information, dependent on others' acceptance of her post-surgical body. These texts discursively produce the unrestored body as unhealthy, a return to well-being contingent on a woman's willingness to wear a prosthesis.

Advertisements for prosthetic devices present the mastectomized body as transient and necessitating concealment. I have shown that prosthesis companies use three dominant themes in advertising which market not only their devices but certain understandings of the post-surgical body. First, an emphasis on the scientific and technological authority of their products ensures a level of safety where women can be assured the prosthesis will not escape from the bra and reveal itself and reveal the truth about their breast amputation. Secondly, advertisements suggest that a restitution of femininity through breast restoration will bring a new and better quality of life. And thirdly, they use metaphors of the restored body as being 'whole', 'complete' and 'natural'. The post-surgical body is framed as being risky, unfeminine, unnatural, incomplete and determining a poorer quality of life, the prosthesis thus a necessity to ensure harmony between body and self.

However, I argue a discrepancy emerges in the function of the prosthesis as a nexus between body and self. Problems arise when women are confronted with their prosthetisized body and the work that reminds them that they will never 'get back to normal', never regain their pre-operative body. The prosthesis itself becomes representative of what has been physically and emotionally lost through breast cancer and surgery.

Whilst consumer and advertising texts discursively produce the post-surgical body as incomplete and needing to be 'fixed', women perform their mastectomized bodies in this way in everyday practices. The prosthetisized body necessitates constant surveillance and management and is situated as restrictive and requiring high maintenance. In addition it is positioned as a body 'for others' that only distances the reality of the mastectomized body from a woman's sense of who she is as a woman.

5
Breast Reconstruction

Introduction

At each step of the breast cancer trajectory women are confronted with choices: extent of surgery, adjuvant treatment options, whether to reshape their post-surgical body, and if so, how. The mastectomized body is framed as something that is to be temporary, existing as a hiatus until breast restoration decisions are made.

Breast reconstruction does not necessarily take place at the end of the illness experience, instead women are often encouraged to think about it before breast loss occurs. Prior to mastectomy a woman's surgeon may alert her to the feelings of physical and emotional loss that may follow and offer her the opportunity of breast reconstruction. Before discovering for herself what breast loss may mean, treatment decision making is tailored to hypothetical concerns, leaving enough skin and nipple to make reconstruction easier (for the surgeon) or choosing a mastectomy and reconstruction rather than removing only the affected site for better aesthetic result. In addition the remaining breast may be lifted, shaped, implanted or reduced to match the new breast. From the outset, women are urged to cover up their post-surgical body.

This chapter examines the impact of breast reconstruction on the status of the mastectomized body. For many women who have had a breast amputated, the option of breast reconstruction signals a sense of hope of regaining lost femininity, sexuality and normalcy. In an analysis of five women's accounts of surgical reconstruction I explore the construction of choice and its implications for the post-surgical body. This study demonstrates that while the expectation of regaining two-breastedness prevails, many mastectomized women are unable to rene-gotiate a 'complete' body.

Up to 50 per cent of women seek reconstruction following mastectomy. There are a number of different surgical options available depending on the woman's age, extent of mastectomy, aesthetic priorities and the expertise and operative preference of the surgeon. There are two basic kinds of breast reconstruction, those which involve artificial substances (implants) and those using the woman's own tissue. Either can be done at the time of mastectomy or any number of years afterwards.

Implants

Breast reconstruction using an implant is considered less invasive of the two major reconstructive techniques. A silicone or saline implant can be inserted behind or in front of the pectoral muscle and the skin sewn together producing a bulge. Alternatively a saline implant can be inserted by expander. In this procedure a balloon expander is inserted beneath the skin and chest muscle. Through a tiny valve mechanism buried beneath the skin, the surgeon will periodically inject a salt-water solution to gradually fill the expander over several weeks or months. When the skin is sufficiently stretched, saline is let out until it is of equal size to the natural breast and potentially results in a more natural effect. While problems with silicone gel implants have been well documented[1] they are consistently promoted as feeling more real and having more weight than saline implants. Problems with implants in general include the risk of them fracturing and leaking and the reconstruction completely collapsing, and the fact that the implant will not lose or gain weight with the recipient.

Flap methods

Options which use a woman's own body to reconstruct the breast are more invasive with much longer operation and recovery times. These techniques involve the removal of skin, muscle and fat from another part of the body, such as the stomach, back or hip, and its transfer to the chest wall. Two of the most popular flap procedures are the TRAM (transverse rectus abdominis muscle) flap, using the abdominal muscle and the latissimus dorsi flap, which combines the use of skin and muscle from the back to cover a saline implant and thereby reconstruct the breast. Although mesh is fitted where the muscle is removed, women can experience subsequent weakness in that area. These types of operations carry greater risks as more of the body is being affected and it will involve more scarring. Nipples can be reconstructed with skin from the labia, inner thigh or other site at any time after the breast reconstruction, or alternatively they can be tattooed on.

Feminist debates about cosmetic surgery

The question of whether women freely choose to have cosmetic surgery or whether they are 'duped by a male-dominated beauty system'[2] has been widely debated within feminist circles. Parker (1995) argues that women may indeed make informed and competent decisions to receive breast implants but that the cultural construction of beauty may undermine women's autonomy by influencing the evaluation of surgical candidates and risk disclosure during informed consent. Similarly, Pauly Morgan (1991) argues that pressures on women to conform to 'Baywatch' standards and undergo cosmetic surgery, combined with the conceptualisation of their body as raw material to be shaped and pruned, opens them to exploitation by men wielding power. She argues that there is a 'paradox of choice' whereby it looks as if women are making their own decisions and cultivating their own bodies, whereas in fact their bodies are being colonised by men. She suggests that we live in a culture that increasingly requires women to 'purchase femininity through submission to cosmetic surgeons and their magic knives'.[3]

Gagné and McGaughey (2002) conclude that individual women may choose to resist or rebel against hegemonic standards of feminine beauty, and women who elect cosmetic mammoplasty exercise agency, but do so within the confines of hegemonic gender norms. In contrast, Davis (1994) emphasizes women's agency in choosing cosmetic surgery arguing that they are knowledgeable and responsible and no 'more duped by the feminine-beauty system than women who do not see cosmetic surgery as a remedy to their problems with their appearance'.[4] Cosmetic surgery can be seen as both a symptom and a solution, oppression and liberation all at once.[5]

As a procedure which is not medically necessary in the treatment of breast cancer, reconstruction is an aesthetic practice. Categorising breast reconstruction in this way has major financial implications for the women who seek it. A surgeon or general practitioner must deem the operation 'medically necessary' for it to be eligible for a Medicare rebate or coverage by a private health insurer.[6] The women in this study had mixed understandings of whether or not breast reconstruction was in fact covered by Medicare. However, surgeons do not necessarily disclose the information. Women described surgeons actively discouraging reconstruction as a public patient because of potentially long waiting lists, and being made feel their only option was to take out expensive private health cover. As a medically unnecessary procedure which has no effect on morbidity or mortality, breast reconstruction remains a largely unexplored issue in women's studies or sociology of health and the body.

Comfort, control or conformity?

Substantial contributions from the traditions of health services research focuses on identity, emotion and quality of life after breast cancer[7] and more specifically on post-mastectomy decision making and attitudes towards prostheses and reconstruction.[8] These studies code breast reconstruction positively as the ultimate goal for women who have undergone mastectomy and the preferred option if fears about possible complications are alleviated. One study suggests women who 'refuse' reconstruction are physically, psychologically and socially poorer than those who seek it.[9] Other writers suggest increased psychological distress the longer the delay after mastectomy.[10] Literature written by surgeons themselves gives the distinct impression *all* mastectomy patients want reconstruction and would have it but for the potential financial burden and further health risks.[11]

Unlike conventional psychosocial research, most feminist analyses situate breast reconstruction as a form of social control, as perpetuating stereotypes of women and their bodies, and as a façade of recovery from a breast cancer crisis.

Ferguson (2000) argues breast reconstruction is used to promote conformity to societal norms of beauty and femininity. Situated as an aspect of the broader medicalization of women's breasts, she states that women with breasts that differ from the norm in size, shape and number are considered deviant. Following Ferguson, I argue that reconstruction perpetuates the pressures on women to realign themselves with the ideal female body. Similarly, Kasper (1995) argues that each woman faces a body in opposition to societal ideals of how the female body should look, an opposition from which the medical profession is only too willing to promise an escape.

The history of the surgical management of breast cancer illustrates it as a powerful mechanism of control over women's bodies and their experience of them.[12] The power of surgeons is heightened by the prestige of surgery within the medical hierarchy, the extremely small number of female surgeons, and the fact that the woman concerned is often experiencing a life threatening condition which can heighten existing dependency and incapacity.[13] Davis (1998) argues that plastic surgery is the most 'gendered' of all medical specialities, as it 'expresses and reproduces the gender symbolism which has men doing the operating while women are the recipients of the surgery, the objects to be operated on'.[14]

Ferguson suggests that breast augmentation and reconstruction are used as forms of social control over women arguing that the specific cultural constraints under which women choose them are grounded in 'the institutional agents of medicalization and social control rather than women's individual agency'.[15] Ferguson examines the role of the American Society of Plastic and Reconstructive Surgeons (ASPRS), the American Medical Association (AMA) and breast implant manufacturers, illustrating how each profits from the medicalization of women's breasts, reinforcing the ideology that women's breasts are diseased or defective.

The positioning of reconstruction as a necessity for mastectomized women, and as the only alternative to prostheses, demands a rethinking of the framing of the post-surgical body. As a beacon of hope, breast reconstruction is situated as the final step in realigning body and self.[16] In what follows I examine the accounts of five women; one who was booked in to have the procedure done and four others who have had the reconstruction. I examine the reasons they give for seeking out the procedure, their experiences of finding the right surgeon, and how they feel towards their reconstructed post-surgical body.

All of these women describe something missing about their sense of self following mastectomy. Not all directly point to what is wrong with their changed bodies and lives, but they can articulate how reconstruction will positively change them. Reconstructive surgery is described as having the potential to restore femininity, normalcy, a complete sense of self and as eliminating the daily hassles of prostheses. With breast reconstruction available, they are unable to imagine a complete body without two breasts.

Reasons for seeking reconstruction

Stephanie, 53, is a primary school teacher in Canberra. Prior to her diagnosis she was also studying social work part-time. She has been divorced from the father of her three children for many years and has recently begun a new relationship with a man she plans to marry later in the year. Stephanie was diagnosed with breast cancer nearly a year before our interview took place, and had a mastectomy followed by chemotherapy. In addition she is on a five-year course of tamoxifen. Stephanie has been to see a number of plastic surgeons and has now settled on who will do the operation. Her reconstruction is booked in for the end of the month in which I interviewed her.

Stephanie describes the disconnection she feels to the self she knew prior to her illness:

> I mean I was a very feminine woman, and I used to have this long blonde hair and I just thought why should I have to put all that away. If there's a chance that I can feel me again, to me I'm just not me . . . and I know that's a lot due to medication and what not, but I just felt like well I'd been mutilated. Well, I don't like using that word, it's not really the one I'm looking for, but just didn't feel complete.

Bodily changes brought about by cancer treatment affect the outward symbols of Stephanie's femininity, something she describes as a definitive part of her self. Unable to recognize her new corporeality she seeks what she considers the only alternative to 'putting away' her past self – reconstruction.

She talks about her reaction to seeing her mastectomy:

> Oh I could look at it uh, ugh, first up I looked, it was huge, and I burst out crying, straight away, and oh, put it away again didn't want to look at it. But then you know you've got to accept it I suppose, but then I thought no, I'm not accepting this. There is no way I am accepting this and I am having another boob there as soon as possible. I will not accept it, and I still won't accept it, and I'm having a reconstruction done as soon as possible. The doctor left extra skin there for reconstruction and I've just been to see two surgeons, to see what they've got to say, two plastic surgeons. And I've just been tossing up which operation I'd have.

For Stephanie the only avenue available to her in order to 'feel me again' is to have a reconstruction. She refuses to renegotiate her changed body and instead positions the relocation of her femininity as dependent on plastic surgery.

Stephanie describes her expectations of the operation:

> I'll feel like, yes, I'll feel really feminine again. And that's important to me. I know that's, I am one of four girls in my family, and they're pretty flat the other three [laugh]. I've got enough for all [laugh]. So, they can't really relate. I mean I've had these since I was about 10 years old. I grew very early.

Stephanie's breasts, and the feminine self they symbolize, are a vital part of who she is. Having decided to go through with the operation, she is now thinking about the type of reconstruction to have:

> I just wish I had known to have it done at the time [of mastectomy]...
> Now that I know, if anything happens to my other breast, I will have
> it done at the same time. I was going to have the big operation, what
> they call the Trans Flap [TRAM Flap], from the stomach, but they
> take a muscle up as well you know. But it was a very attractive
> thought because I've had this horrible stomach for years because I had
> three caesarians, and I've got these scars. So he [the surgeon] said he
> could get rid of all of that and give me a tummy tuck and I thought
> whoa, yes you gotta be happy with that! But because of the scarring
> there's not enough tissue there. So what he's going to have to do is
> use some of that [abdominal tissue], take the muscle from there too,
> but put a prosthesis [implant] in as well. So I have to have both
> done! And the whole idea of having that operation is not to have
> anything foreign in my body. And he said well I haven't got enough
> to make up a breast because your breasts are so dense and bla bla bla.
> And there won't be enough raw tissue. What he said he'll try and do
> is another operation a couple of weeks beforehand and cut off three
> areas to, to see how much survives, and what survives we'll move up,
> and we might get a bit more. But, it became less and less attractive as
> time went on...So I've decided that I will go with the prosthesis
> [implant] way, just have the expander and all the rest of it. But I know
> that's not going to be the same, I know that's going to sit out higher
> and all that sort of stuff. But for all intents and purposes, wearing
> clothing, it's going to be good. But it really will just feel normal
> again and look a lot more normal than it does.

The surgeon offers Stephanie hope, being able to transform her 'horrible stomach' into a new breast. The wondrous description she gives of this new body quickly diminishes as she articulates the technicality of the procedure: transplant of raw tissues, accepting a foreign object into her body, bits being cut off and then seeing which bits survive. The potential breast shifts from being a site of femininity to something that is 'for all intents and purposes'. Stephanie describes the reconstructed breast as ultimately enabling normalcy, she will *look* and *feel* more normal again.

Margaret, 51, is married and is a lab technician at a university in Canberra. She was diagnosed at the age of 47 and had chemotherapy and a mastectomy. She had a saline implant by expander six months prior to our interview.

Initially Margaret was prevented from having reconstructive surgery because she could not afford it. This obstacle fueled her depression and her mother stepped in to help. Margaret talks about why she sought a reconstruction:

> I wanted to have a reconstruction, I, um, a couple of women I know through Bosom Buddies had reconstructions, and they seemed quite happy. I was told I could have one in the public health system, but that is not correct, and it's something people should be aware of. Most plastic surgeons will not [do it] if you're a public patient, they'll just close the book. So I gave up on the idea. But my Mother, last year, was aware that my depression was getting worse, and she gave me the money to have a reconstruction. So that was really, really great.
>
> I've never had a very good, my self image isn't very good, but then after this happened I thought, well you didn't have anything to complain about before. I don't know, everybody's self image is different. Some women don't really care – I see women with drooping breasts who don't even wear a bra, and I think you know, it's just the same isn't it really. It's an individual thing.

Reconstruction is positioned as the only available mechanism to overcome her poor self-image. Contrasting her body prior to illness to her post-surgical one allows no space to accept her mastectomized body in any form. Instead she speaks of reconstruction as a solution to poor self-image both prior to surgery and after.

Petrea, 49, is a public servant in Canberra and a married mother of three teenage children. Her husband is 'into computers' and they live in a modest house in the city's north. Petrea was diagnosed when she was 39 and had a lumpectomy, mastectomy, chemotherapy, radiotherapy and was on a five-year course of tamoxifen. She had a saline implant one year after her mastectomy, which had to be removed some time afterwards due to it rupturing. She then had a Transverse Rectus Abdominal Muscle (TRAM) flap reconstruction.

Petrea decided before her mastectomy that she wanted reconstruction, and was thus left with a sac of skin ready to be filled. Petrea describes her first looking at her mastectomy:

> It was pretty horrible. I didn't want to look at it. I woke up with a great bandage over the whole thing. And then only when they took

me in to have a shower at the hospital I got to see it there. The difference with my mastectomy which I think is quite unusual is that I still had the nipple because the surgeon wanted to make it as easy as possible for reconstruction and seemed to think that was okay. So it looked pretty horrible at the time. The skin was all still there, it was saggy, but the actual breast was taken out of the middle of it.

I always wanted to have it [reconstruction]. And in the long run a lot of it was just because when I get up in the morning I like to just pull clothes on and just go. And so it just became...it was back to normal again you know, just put on a bra without having to fiddle around with anything you know sort of check that you didn't look too bad flat on one side. And so that was one of my reasons.

Fiddling with her prosthesis was a constant reminder of her breast loss and drew attention to the necessity of perpetual self-monitoring. Petrea was comfortable not wearing a prosthesis but the cosmetic result of her mastectomy positioned her body as unfinished and so felt she must get the operation.

Anna is 50 and a retired school teacher. She is now a non-fiction writer and devotes a small amount of time to a national breast cancer support and advocacy group. She lives in country NSW, is married to a GP and has four adult children. Her first diagnosis of breast cancer at 40 resulted in a mastectomy and chemotherapy. Seven years later she had cancer in her other breast and had her second mastectomy. Anna had a bilateral reconstruction at the time of her second mastectomy, a decision that her husband strongly opposed. He thought it was 'too big an operation' to have at one time, but in the end supported her choice.

Anna talks about how she felt towards her breasts before her mastectomies:

My breasts were beautiful [laugh]. They were the only decent part of me and here they were being taken away. I mean some people have horrible breasts, and good legs and a good bum or whatever, but I was a breasts woman. They were definitely a part of me, um, and they didn't even sag, after four kids breastfed, like they should have. That's probably why I found the need to reconstruct them, I don't know...And um, taking away your breasts is like taking away a major part of your sexuality, now you don't necessarily have to be acting upon that sexuality, it's just how you view yourself. And if that's damaged, you want to make it whole again. It's not just a lump of fat on the front of you, um, there's something more about your self-image. Something in a person.

Anna identifies herself as a 'breasts woman' locating her breasts as a vital part of her sense of self. She situates her body and self as inextricably linked, as a 'whole'. She draws on a discourse which frames women's mastectomized bodies as physically, sexually and emotionally incomplete. At the same time she positions the restoration of body and self as simple, breast reconstruction simultaneously bringing back the physical, the sexual and the emotional.

> Mind you, I'm very glad too, that all I've had to have cut off is something superficial and not something deep and I don't have to have a colostomy bag, or something like that . . . If you'd asked me about it, I would have said no way having a breast off would have really worried me, it have been a nuisance, not that fond of my breasts anyway, um, you've got two, you can do without one, marriage is solid, it doesn't matter to you, there is more to a marriage than that you know. I would have thought all those things. Nothing, nothing at all prepared me for the actual feeling.

Anna situates her breasts as dispensable and replaceable, contradicting the 'whole' she describes earlier. This disjuncture highlights the complexity of breast loss as Anna recollects how she thought she would feel towards her breast loss and the reality.

Gemma, 33, is single and divorced a couple of years ago. When I first met Gemma she was a bank manager but resigned during the course of her illness. Her mother was diagnosed with breast cancer five years ago and Gemma believes the stress of that combined with her divorce triggered the growth of her own tumour. She lives in a new development on the outskirts of Canberra in NSW. I spoke to Gemma eight months after her diagnosis, prior to her breast implant, and again two months later, after she had the reconstruction. She had a mastectomy with no adjuvant treatment, but takes mineral enhanced water in the hope of warding off recurrences. Gemma is the secretary of Bosom Buddies and started a young women's group within the organization.

Gemma's mother's experience of mastectomy directly affected her own decision making regarding reconstruction:

> My mother has had breast cancer, and she has had her right breast removed, and I just thought, Mum's always had a prosthesis, and I know the difficulties she's had with a prosthesis, and I didn't want to be prepared to put up with a prosthesis, and I wanted to be reasonably normal again. I didn't want to be different. It was so hard for me

to accept the decision that had been made about the mastectomy, I felt that reconstruction was an avenue for me to feel reasonably normal again. And it was suggested by my surgeon, in the early stages as well, which was really good.

For Gemma, the prosthesis represents an obstacle to a return to normal, thoughts which are confirmed by her surgeon.

Speaking with her before the reconstruction, Gemma talks about her concerns:

Just that it's not going to work, um if it doesn't work that's ok, it's just something I'll have to deal with at the time, um and at the end of the day I'll just go back to being what I am now, which is fine, um, but yeah, that it's not going to work. And going through more surgery is, I'm not looking forward to having more surgery. I've only had a couple of operations, but the process that I've been through, particularly with the initial needle biopsy that I had and the wire into my breast when I had the lumpectomy, it was pretty awful, very confronting, really awful situation that I went through. So yeah, having more surgery.

To be relegated to 'what I am now' is to be different and abnormal. Gemma positions her mastectomized body as unacceptable, something she is unable to renegotiate alone:

I'm not in a relationship with someone, where somebody's there to say you still look gorgeous, you're still wonderful and all that sort of stuff. I have only got me to look in the mirror each day and think, oh [sigh] I'm different. And I don't know whether it's ok or not. To me it's not ok. Although the scar is pretty terrific! [laugh]. I mean the surgeon has done a really great job [laugh] and it's really nice and neat and even and it's just healing up beautifully, um, but I think if you had someone there saying you look terrific – well my friends tell me I look terrific and that sort of thing, it's still just, yeah.

Gemma seeks permission to accept her body as normal and 'ok' without a breast.

In these accounts all five women suggest breast reconstruction is a pragmatic alternative to prostheses. However, it is simultaneously presented as being much more than this. Stephanie, Margaret and Gemma depict the operation as enabling a symbolic restoration of femininity, and both

Stephanie and Anna see it as a portal to prior sense of self. In contrast Anna also presents reconstruction as ultimately superficial, as breasts are something which exist almost as an external appendage to the body. Women struggle with their sense of their breasts as part of superficial appearance, and a much more deep-seated sense of their sexuality of which their breasts were a critical part.

Plastic surgeons can have a great influence on a woman's decision to have a reconstruction. In the surgeon–patient encounter the healthy mastectomized body is medicalized as something which needs to be corrected, constructing it as inherently abnormal and incomplete.

The context of breast restoration decision making

At each step of the breast cancer trajectory women are confronted with choices: extent of surgery, adjuvant treatment options and how to reshape their post-surgical body. The mastectomized body is situated as something that is to be temporary, existing as a hiatus until breast restoration decisions are made.

Breast reconstruction does not necessarily take place at the end of the illness experience, instead women are encouraged to think about it before breast loss occurs. Prior to mastectomy a woman's surgeon may alert her to the feelings of physical and emotional loss that may follow and offer her the opportunity of breast reconstruction. Before discovering for herself what breast loss may mean, treatment decision making is tailored to hypothetical concerns, leaving enough skin and nipple to make reconstruction easier (for the surgeon) or choosing a mastectomy and reconstruction rather than removing only the affected site for better aesthetic result. In addition the non-diseased breast may be lifted, shaped, implanted or reduced to match the new breast. From the outset, women are urged to cover up their post-surgical body.

Margaret describes her experience of finding the right surgeon:

> The surgeons are like car salesman as far as I'm concerned, they're out there to sell their product. Most of them aren't interested in your health, once they know you've had cancer that subject doesn't come up...I did shop around though. The first one just closed his book when he realized I didn't have the money, and he said I'll have to put you on the waiting list, it will take forever, it's not worth it...He took a photograph of me, without the face of course, but I felt really uncomfortable about that. And he was, you know, flashing photographs up on the screen of all these peoples before and after, oh

[sigh], I just thought, how awful, he was basically showing me his work of art! He basically said you can put your name down, but you'll be waiting ten years. Then another one I went to, he was a real car salesman, I mean he stood there while I got undressed, and he was going to turn me into Pamela Anderson by the time he'd finished with me, and that's not why I was there.

Breast reconstruction is a product surgeons sell. The profit incentive is highlighted in the surgeons refusal to treat Margaret as a public patient. Viewing the faceless images of previous surgery, Margaret is left feeling objectified and uncomfortable. Like the first surgeon, the second one she visits similarly situates Margaret as a template from which he will work his 'art', transforming her into a whole new woman:

[H]e was showing me pictures, and he was very proud of what he had done, and he wasn't concerned about me and my breast reconstruction, he wanted to do the other one and even them up, and I could do this and I could do that, and I thought that's not what I'm here for, and I didn't go back to him.

Her body is medicalized further as her healthy breast is situated as needing to be altered. She describes the surgeon as not being concerned with her as a person or the actual surgery she wanted to be done, instead she is an endless set of technical options for the surgeon to perfect.

Margaret consulted a third surgeon, whom she decides to have perform the surgery:

He didn't have any pictures. But he does have a very good reputation and so I trusted him. And I was happy with him. He was very, very concerned about my health, between the two operations, he was very concerned about infection and things like that.

Choosing a saline expander required Margaret to attend a number of follow up consultations:

He [the surgeon] was very concerned about whether I was happy about it or not. Because he had to choose what size to put in, and as I was with most things, I was halfway between one size and another, and so he chose the smaller one, and I suppose on the operating table they must have to sit you up and see how they [the breasts] measure. So when I went back after that, he said was I happy with the size, and I said yes, and he said phew, because we were a bit worried.

On the operating table Margaret's unconscious body is propped up and her new breast judged for its appropriate size and position. Margaret talks about how she felt afterwards:

Well it wasn't that sore actually, it's not as bad as I thought. I was expecting it to be a lot sorer. The tissue expander that they put in is quite big and round and it had a little valve on the side where they add the extra saline, but in fact in some respects I wish I'd left that in because it was a little bit bigger than this prosthesis [implant], and because my scar is across the top of the breast, I actually had a better cleavage with the expander because it was more round and it filled it out more. But it wasn't as comfortable, and there was that valve there, which you could feel. But some people actually leave that in.

For Margaret, the process of breast reconstruction began with the decision she could no longer tolerate the prosthesis. Although initially contemplating nipple restoration, she says 'that's just because I was all caught up in it. But I'm used to it now, the way that it is, and I don't know that I'll bother.' Margaret is now able to accept her body the way it is, albeit without a nipple. At the end of our interview Margaret describes her breast as not looking or feeling like the natural one, but to others it looks normal. She describes her self-image and self-esteem as explicitly dependent on others perception of her body, something she feels is threatened by women who reveal their mastectomy scar or reconstructed breasts publicly.

Gemma talks about what she looks for in a surgeon:

Um, that I'm comfortable with them, that they show care, and they show that they care about me and what I'm going to look like at the end of the day. One particular surgeon that I saw he really only promoted one type of surgery, he was really quite offensive, quite arrogant, and made me feel [pause] quite degraded... He was talking about a TRAM flap operation, which I feel is quite devastating and quite a big operation for some one of my age. He had a look at my tummy, and thought that there was more there than I needed, and I've still got a little bit of breast tissue left, not much, but he was very matter of fact about the fact that you know, you've had a mastectomy you've got nothing there. Um, so he was really quite rough, and I wasn't really needing that at that time. Um, I've gone with two surgeons that have been suggested to me by my breast surgeon, so I've really gone with his recommendations rather than done my own research, but I've felt really comfortable with what he's done, um, and his support and that with me, so I sort of trust, I've been trusting him in his advice about who I should be seeing in this next step.

Gemma feels degraded by the surgeon who objectifies her flesh. His insensitivities to her body image and his offensive manner mean she seeks an alternative opinion. Discussion with the surgeon includes the possibility of doing something to her remaining breast:

It was assumed it was going to be the same size as the other breast, I haven't really spoken much about doing anything with the right breast, only up until my last appointment. That's when I started talking to him about anything that could be done with the right breast because the left breast, or the reconstructed breast is going to be different. So I just wanted him to talk a little bit more about you know, what can you do to make the size look the same, or around about the same shape. Because if you have the reconstructed breast, and you leave the other breast as is, you are going to have a difference, because of ageing processes.

Because of my age and because I'm small in size an implant was the best way to go as well. And I've got those other surgical options down the track, because you know the TRAM Flap is the final thing, but at least I've still got those options down the track anyway...because with implants over a period of time they can become hard, so while some women can have them for 20 or 30 years, other women only have them for five or six. But he was just so easy to talk to, he made me feel like a person not like a surgical option. And he's made me feel quite comfortable with myself and quite beautiful about the whole thing all the way through. He's just been so special, he's really, really lovely.

Her surgeon suggests a small implant in the remaining breast to give a similar shape. Although initially deciding to have this done, she had changed her mind when I spoke with her before the operation. This decision is based around the possible interference it may have when she has mammograms.

Gemma is resigned to the fact that this reconstruction may not be the 'final thing' as implants have a short life expectancy. In addition she faces further surgery in the future, perhaps when her body is more suited to the TRAM flap operation.

While Margaret's and Gemma's surgeons are men who do not make them feel like 'surgical options', their descriptions of the operation shift from being about restoring normalcy and femininity to acquiring the right drop and symmetry. The healthy mastectomized body is situated as an oxymoron by plastic surgeons, the remaining breast needing to be filled out and evened up to match the other. As a next step in the breast cancer trajectory, concern for their health is absent. Instead the focus is on remoulding the woman's body to surgeon's ideals. However, in this process women are enthusiastic and complicit – it is also *their* ideal.

Reconstructing the self

Kasper argues that breast reconstruction fails to meet the expectations of the majority of women, suggesting a 'disjuncture between socially imposed expectations for women and women's own experience of recovery and well being' (1995: 216). Margaret, Petrea, Gemma and Anna talk about how they feel towards their reconstructed breast and its effect on their sense of self.

Margaret sought a reconstruction in the hope it would improve her self-image and realign her body and self as 'normal'. After the surgery she says:

> I felt great. Yeah. It was just so nice to go out, I went straight out and bought some new bras, because I hadn't bought any bras, I'd just lost interest. Every time I went into underwear stores, I got depressed. You know, they were all low cut, nice bras, and I had to wear these high tight ones, so I went straight out and bought some new bras.

The surgery enables Margaret to *do* femininity – to wear nice sexy bras. Previously she was unable to wear such low-cut bras as they would not contain the prosthesis. The prosthesis restricted her choices of lingerie. She goes on:

> There are no reminders that I've had cancer. I felt, after I realized how depressed I had been I realized that I had to have it. I have some friends, and they would never have it done, but it's just different, and the way you feel is different . . . But the breast doesn't look like a breast, it doesn't have a nipple, and it doesn't look like the other breast. But in a bra it's good, and it's a lot more comfortable, rather than a

prosthesis that's hot and sweaty, and you have to wash it – it's a lot of work. And after a while, I just got so tired of putting it in bras and watching if I had to lean down, and it's just more convenient.

Margaret attributes the necessity of her reconstruction to worsening depression, the reconstruction being the only avenue which could improve her self-image. Although she suggests she has no reminders of cancer, the reconstructed breast, which looks and feels different, is a very real reminder of what she has been through. Ultimately, her reconstructed breast is more 'convenient' and the only alternative to the hassles of prostheses and poor body image.

Petrea describes the reconstruction she had one year after her mastectomy, shortly before being posted overseas for her husband's work.

The reconstruction that I had was a ... they pump it up with saline, and then it is supposed to be replaced later on with a silicone or a different sort of saline implant. So I had that done and that took quite a long time because you have to go back every week and have some more saline injected into it until it gets to be twice as big as the real one. And then they take some of it out. It's supposed to make it fall in a natural way. And also I had a muscle moved from the back to the front to help and it was because of the blood flow or something ... And when it got to the same size it was good, and then it got to be larger and it was a bit much to take. But then it was back to being reasonably natural after that. I felt good about it ... but I have no sensation at all. I never have.

Petrea's reconstructed breast is situated as not real. She has no feeling in it although it appears 'normal'.

But then when I went overseas, we went to Ireland, and I had a mammogram there and they insisted on doing a mammogram on the prosthetic breast and they broke the implant. And so then I had to have another reconstruction – I didn't really notice it until about a week later and it was suddenly deflated – I went to a plastic surgeon there and he said that I really needed to have it out. And then he didn't really want to put another implant in, he thought the best would be to do a TRAM flap reconstruction, and I'd put on so much [weight] by that time. And that has been really good ... And it was sewed up through the skin and sort of popped out ... it's actually a bit better than the saline implant because that used to move around a lot more under my arm...Lying down it would go right down under there [pointing to underarm] and I'd be completely flat. Now the reconstructed one is up higher [than the natural breast] and it stays like that. It looks similar, very similar in a bra but otherwise if I am just wearing a T-shirt or something, no.

The deflation of Petrea's breast highlights just how unreal it is. Her subsequent reconstruction leaves the breast sitting differently and still with no sensation. For a woman who was happy to live without the prosthesis for a year after her mastectomy she is blasé about the surgery. To Petrea it is simply practical.

Gemma describes waking up after her reconstruction:

I was in a corset, an elasticized corset, so I couldn't see anything, but I could see that I had shape. And it was the next morning when the doctor came around to visit me that I could see what had happened. He unzipped me and undid the corset and all that kind of thing and then I saw that I had shape. And that was really lovely. I wasn't really emotional about it or anything at that stage, it, because it was really quite swollen and quite different to the other side. It was really different at that point in time, but I was really pleased with it. It wasn't until I was driving one morning and I felt it move, like it just sort of, then to me it felt natural, and that was when I cried. That was when I got really upset. But that was just because I finally, it finally sort of felt like I had something natural again.

In a scene reminiscent of the Victorian era, the powerful manly doctor unzips Gemma's corset revealing his masterpiece. She is unconditionally pleased, even without having seen it, just seeing the 'shape' is enough. Unfortunately for Gemma, a couple of weeks after her reconstruction it is apparent there are problems with the implant which means another operation:

I'm one of the one in 500 or one in 1000 that you have problems. The problem with mine is, I don't know whether it's because of my age and because of the muscle structure, but my pectoral muscles pulled the implant up. That only happened over a period of a few weeks and over time it probably would have eventually naturally come back down into place, but my surgeon decided to intervene now because he was looking for the perfect result and he wanted to intervene with another operation. And that operation was probably only half an hour, but it was another general anesthetic – that's four in ten months – and he actually had to physically pull the implant down two and a half inches, so the muscle had pulled it quite away. And the implant had actually rotated as well, so he had to put it back into place and pull it down. And with the particular implant that I've got, it's in a tear shape, so it had to sit right.

Gemma assumes responsibility, her body having betrayed this new source of femininity and normalcy. Her muscles pull it up high near her collar bone. Although she thinks it would naturally come back down and integrate with the rest of her body, the surgeon is not prepared to wait in pursuit of the 'perfect result'. She describes how her new breast feels:

It's, because of the mastectomy a lot of the tissue was taken away that had nerves and that in it, but you can still feel touch, like the sensitivity is not there, but you can still feel touch. I'm three weeks away from my last operation now, and the swelling's gone down quite a bit and it's starting to soften up, so it's not like a hard, round ball anymore it's starting to soften up a bit more and feel a bit more natural. And I'm fitting into a bra and that sort of thing as well. I mean, whilst everybody's different, to just go and be fitted into a nice bra again it's really, really lovely. I mean lingerie isn't the be all and end all but it's all still to do with having a mastectomy, there's a lot of loss of femininity, or I felt that I lost a lot of my feminine side. So just getting back into bras again and having the shape there it's really good... Whilst it looks different and that sort of thing, I think just the feeling of having the shape there again and being able to wear t-shirts with confidence and being able to wear the clothes that I used to wear, because I haven't been able to feel comfortable wearing all my clothes. Not that I have a lot of low cut clothing or anything like that, but with the prosthesis it was really difficult – fitting it into a bra, making sure it stayed in the bra, swimming and that sort of thing, it's just, it's not an issue anymore, it's taken away so many issues.

Whilst the removal of a prosthesis may minimize the physical effect of breast loss, the emotional consequences of breast cancer and surgery do not disappear:

But [having had breast cancer] does creep up on you still from time to time, and I don't know that I'll ever get closure as such with having been through what I've been through. Because I think the things that I've mentioned about femininity and sexuality being taken away, yeah there's still a couple of small bridges. The physical doesn't just replace, whilst for me it feels beautiful and reasonably natural, and I laugh about it with friends...

I asked whether she would recommend reconstruction to other women:

Absolutely. Yep, yep... On the basis of not having to worry about the prosthesis anymore. Having the shape and being comfortable in wearing just about anything again. Even if I wanted to wear something low cut, which I wouldn't, but if I did I could easily. And it was an easy operation, you know it wasn't a painfully traumatic operation.

Three weeks from her last operation, Gemma is positive and enthusiastic about the results. Although she now says the procedure was 'easy' she endured four large operations (two to remove the cancer) in the space of 10 months and had noted previously what an ordeal it had been on her body.

Like Margaret, Gemma's reconstructed breast enables a doing of femininity through having more variety of lingerie to wear. However, Gemma admits there are still a few 'small bridges' to cross when dealing with issues of lost femininity and sexuality through breast loss. While she describes her reconstructed body as more normal and 'reasonably' natural she is matter-of-fact about the limitations of simply replacing the physical. Petrea describes more realistic expectations she had of her reconstruction, as alleviating the daily body work the prosthesis necessitated. Although Margaret and Gemma present reconstruction as a source of femininity and normalcy, they too situate it as an ultimately pragmatic solution to negate the hassles of prostheses.

While most women in this study spoke about the availability of reconstruction positively, one woman offered an alternative interpretation. Anna decided to have both breasts reconstructed at the same time she had her second mastectomy. However, there were complications during the operation as the blood vessels fail to connect. She ends up in surgery five times in the following week and her reconstructed breasts become partially gangrenous. Here is part of the dialogue we had about her unsuccessful reconstruction:

[W]hereas I thought I'd be having a reconstruction to try to regain some sort of self-confidence in my body, I ended up with a lot more scarring... And I was just one of the unlucky ones, the person was brilliant, I don't have a problem with him, but it was just one side took and the other one didn't. So I ended up more damaged by the reconstruction than if I'd been flat chested.

SC: So what happened after the five operations?

I was at death's door. It was a reconstruction of my vanity I suppose if you want to put it like that . . . it was such an assault on my system, everything went wrong.

SC: And are your breasts reconstructed now?

No. I left them half way through. Everything's healed and I've got nice rounded breasts of approximately the same size. But no nipples, which is wonderful because I can go out in the coldest air! I've come to grips with um, body damage. Probably took back some of the, of what I should have come to grips with in the first mastectomy. But the damaged body, I probably didn't come to grips with until after I had all this done.

SC: Why after that?

I had no choice. You see I always had the option of reconstruction, when I didn't have a breast, I always had the option there. I knew if I wanted to be whole again, I could, right? And maybe that had something to do with it, but after the gangrene business for example . . . instead of coming home and showing my husband these beautiful pert breasts, I was getting him to take gangrene off . . . so probably that caused me to come to grips with a lot of things altogether. That incident. It was really what I should have gone through after the first mastectomy.

Anna talks about the hope of regaining some self-confidence in her body after the reconstruction, but instead ending up more 'damaged'. This damage has both physical and emotional implications. For Anna the failed reconstruction of her breasts, and herself, means that she has to come to grips with her post-surgical body and self. While the *option* of reconstruction, of becoming 'whole again', was available to her, she felt that she could not or did not deal with her post-surgical body in the way that she should have. The possibility of reconstruction symbolized a sense of hope, in that if she wanted to regain normality and complete womanhood she could. While that choice was available it meant that she did not come to terms with her body or who she was, a woman affected by the consequences of breast cancer: a woman whose body was damaged by having a breast amputated. Breast reconstruction as a point of recovery is revealed to be false.

Anna talks about the surgeon who did the operation:

> The plastic surgeon's beautiful, he keeps sending me messages to go back and see him. He wants to finish off, he's not happy that I haven't got perfect breasts now...like all his other patients have. But it was such a trauma with everything going wrong that I haven't been prepared to line up voluntarily to get it tidied up. I will one day, probably, but I don't, um, I know it's only really minor to finish it off, but I'm quite, I think I've come to grips with being damaged through that incident, so it doesn't worry me that my breasts aren't normal any more.

The surgeon situates Anna's post-surgical body as messy and incomplete. Even though Anna has accepted her 'body damage' she feels a certain obligation to the surgeon, to be aligned as 'perfect' like his other patients.

I asked Anna if she would recommend it to other women:

> No I wouldn't recommend it to anybody. Not because of the medical aspect, and what went wrong, but because I think in most cases, it indicates that the woman hasn't come to grips with who she is.

Conclusion

Women seeking reconstructions hold a number of contradictory expectations. While women suggest that reconstruction will restore lost femininity, sexuality and normalcy, I argue that in most cases it is not the procedure that enables this but the elimination of the hassles of prostheses. In contrast to the complete sense of self they expected to regain through reconstruction, they articulate a restoration that is simply pragmatic – they are able to wear clothes and lingerie more easily as they do not have to tend to a prosthetisized body. Women described how eliminating prostheses enabled a doing of femininity, sexuality and normalcy through the freedom to wear clothes they felt were unavailable to them previously. However, this raises questions: Can this performance of the post-surgical body be achieved without having to resort to surgical reconstruction? And if so, what mechanisms are available to support and encourage women to do so?

Prior to reconstruction these women describe their bodies as different, abnormal and personally and publicly unacceptable, an interpretation vindicated by the surgeons they visit. Plastic surgeons translate the mastectomized body into a series of surgical options from which the woman and her health are absent. In addition, her natural breast is often medicalized and positioned as needing to be simultaneously 'fixed'.

Unlike psychosocial research which codes reconstruction positively, the small number of feminist analyses situate it as a form of social control, as reproducing stereotypes of women and their bodies and as a façade of recovery from breast cancer. I have argued that the availability of reconstruction signifies a hope that the post-surgical body can be physically restored which in turn will enable a harmony between body and self. However, reconstruction does not restore the body to how it looked or felt prior to illness. Women are left with a breast shape that is still scarred, sits differently to the natural breast, has little or no sensitivity, does not necessarily have a nipple, and often results in scars to other parts of their body. This non-breast appears as a lump of flesh, symbolizing neither the erotic nor maternal of the original breast. In their absence two breasts signified a 'complete' self, embodying normalcy, sexuality and femininity. Although some women described their reconstruction positively, I argue that it is only after the surgery fails to deliver what they expected that they are forced to renegotiate their sense of themselves as women with or without breasts. As Anna said, it was not until the option of reconstruction was no longer available that she was able to come to terms with her maimed body and self.

Many other women for whom reconstruction is still an option remain unable to fully conceptualize a 'whole' self without two breasts. Instead they perform their bodies as abnormal and incomplete by situating reconstruction as the only alternative to the hassles of prostheses and as the source of hope that all can be restored if they had the time and money to do so.

6
Conclusions

Many assumptions are made about women who have a breast amputated. First, they will want all evidence of their breast cancer concealed. Secondly, they will want breast shape restored as soon as possible. Thirdly, this will be done either by wearing a prosthesis or by having the breast or breasts surgically reconstructed.

Breast restoration technologies – prostheses and surgical reconstruction – are a firm component of the breast cancer trajectory. However, women may need to relocate their sense of womanhood after mastectomy without having to submit themselves to further surgery or endure the problems associated with prostheses. The necessity of reconstruction for aesthetic purposes, to make clothes hang better and so on, demands a rethinking of the positioning of the mastectomized body in today's society.

I have examined how the post-surgical body is negotiated, constituted, mobilized and performed by and for women with breast cancer. In paying attention to the ways in which meanings and understandings of the mastectomized body are discursively and materially produced we can begin to see how knowledge is constructed and the implications this knowledge has for the self. Objects, things, words and actions all *perform* the post-surgical body in particular ways and produce frameworks of meaning in which the self is positioned.

Four main themes thread through this book. First, the construction of breast cancer knowledge. Understandings of breast cancer derive from women with breast cancer, medical specialists, breast cancer organizations, and corporations who benefit financially from breast cancer treatment. Feminist scholars have identified the way biomedically defined experiences fall short of lived experiences,[1] the limited number of meanings from which women can choose when trying to make sense of their illness experience[2] and the historical and cultural contexts in which the construction of breast cancer knowledge occurs.[3] While supporting the findings of these researchers, this study makes an important addition to the literature by examining the meanings attributed to the mastectomized body at the intersection of biomedical discourse, breast cancer culture and women's experiences. I note that each woman's experience of her post-surgical body is filled with ambiguity and uncertainty, contradictions and tensions.

The second major theme is the renegotiation of identity during, and as a result of, breast cancer and breast surgery. This study extends previous research findings that reveal the body to be a site of ambiguity and anxiety.[4] I move beyond individual experiences to examine the politics of the choices available to women and what constrains and influences those choices. Such an approach provides a powerful analysis of the decision-making dilemmas facing women after breast cancer and surgery, and the socio-political context in which their decisions about breast restoration are made. I examine the role of breast cancer organizations and challenge the hegemonic breast cancer identity they promote.

The disconnection of body and self is the third major theme of this research. Popular in research in the sociology and psychology of anorexia,[5] self/body dualism has been used to explore notions of an ideal body 'for others' and an embodied corporeality. I apply such notions to explore how 'becoming whole' after mastectomy is a metaphor for recovery where self and body appear in harmony. This exploration brings into question the role of advocacy and support groups in influencing women's decision making regarding breast restoration, something which is revealed to potentially distance a woman's body and sense of self. Women describe a disconnection between the self they knew prior to illness, the self they project to others following breast loss and the self they feel they conceal through use of prostheses. This research makes an original contribution to studies of the self and post-surgical body[6] by examining the medical institutions and prostheses manufacturers who promote and benefit from the disconnecting of the mastectomized body and a woman's sense of who she is as a woman without breasts.

In women's narratives the post-surgical body is situated as a site of ambiguity and uncertainty and as having a distinct lack of fit with dominant notions of how the mastectomized body should look and feel. Although they have negotiated a new sense of self following a breast cancer crisis, this new self is at odds with their changed body. The new identity that has been formed through their breast cancer experience lacks coherence with the corporeal self they simultaneously describe. The tropes which enable the articulation of their mastectomized body and self perform this body within a negative frame, as essentially lacking and necessitating restoration for the sake of others. With no alternative discourse available, positive images and experiences of the post-surgical body cannot be normalized and the dominant narrative of the feminine body is perpetuated. This constitutes the fourth major theme of this book, the silence that pervades the post-surgical body. Thus the stories women tell reproduce breast amputation as something which must necessarily be covered up and spoken about only in terms of lack and concealment. In spite of the multiplicity of feelings and meanings the woman herself may attribute to her changed body, she discursively produces it in accordance with a dominant script that does not allow for individual exploration. Instead the mastectomized body is performed as overwhelmingly unacceptable and conditions the prefigured response of using prostheses or surgical reconstruction.

Mainstream breast cancer culture mobilizes dominant narratives of the post-surgical body reproducing it as unfeminine, desexualized and abnormal. The largely white, middle-class, middle-aged, heterosexual 'sisterhood' of breast cancer advocates promotes an emotional and physical response to breast loss based on hyperfeminine norms. To position oneself outside this frame is precarious. There is virtually no space to develop the movement around acceptance of the mastectomized body. Large-scale fundraising events and constant media attention enable the breast cancer movement to publicly mobilize certain meanings and understandings of the mastectomized body. In events such as the Bosom Buddies fashion parade and 'Field of Women', and in individual encounters newly diagnosed women have with breast cancer volunteers, norms about how the post-surgical body should look and act are constituted in visual representations of the repaired body beautiful. Furthermore, breast cancer culture frames the restoration of heterofeminine aesthetic hegemony as a social obligation. Pink advocacy perpetuates a homogenous response to breast loss and provides limited space for women to consider alternative mechanisms with which to reconceptualize the changed landscape of their post-surgical body.

Pink advocates, the medical profession and cancer organizations promote this discourse through their speech, texts and objects offered to newly diagnosed women. Regardless of how an individual may feel about her breast amputation or whether she has even begun to consider the effect it may have on her sense of self as a woman, she is bombarded with messages that do this work for her. Consumer literature published or endorsed by cancer organizations, and brochures from prosthesis companies, frame the mastectomized body as unhealthy and needing to be corrected. Booklets detailing emotional, sexual and physical rehabilitation following breast cancer and surgery make clear the link between recovery from a breast cancer crisis and the restoration of a 'normal' two-breasted appearance. In these texts women are reduced to a set of physical attributes that signify self-worth and well-being.

Advertisements for prosthetic devices locate femininity, sexuality and normalcy firmly within a two-breasted appearance. Furthermore, these components of a woman's sense of self are positioned as detachable as they are located within an inanimate object – the prosthesis. The prosthesis is thus a nexus between body and self, performing the 'whole woman' when it is worn. However, enacting this 'complete' self in everyday practices reveals that this nexus is unstable as women are confronted with the constant management prostheses require. Women discover not a new 'whole' self and body, rather one that is uncomfortable, risky and requiring high maintenance. Rather than enabling recovery prostheses hinder the process as they act as a constant reminder of the realities of the post-surgical body. Thus as women position their pros-thesis in their bra, constantly check to make sure it is not about to fall out, are unable to appear without it in public or to their partner, and attempt to tolerate any uncomfortable reaction their skin may have to the device, they perform their post-surgical body as incomplete and abnormal. The prosthesis then further distances body from self and reminds them of their loss. Women are thus unable to reconceptualize themselves as fully recovered with or without a prosthesis; instead the only alternative is to eliminate daily hassles by more permanent breast restoration – surgical reconstruction.

Following breast amputation women are presented with two choices: to wear a prosthesis or undergo reconstruction. Breast restoration is assumed to allow a full emotional and physical recovery. For women who have worn prostheses prior to reconstruction, the operation enables freedom from the restrictive tendencies of the prosthetisized body. In the case of women who have the procedure done at the same time as mastectomy, they awake to a lump of flesh that looks and feels nothing like the breast it replaces. Still in the images and representations of the mastectomized body available to them these are the mechanisms available with which to deal with their altered corporeality. By constructing hope, these technologies are a way of ordering the chaos of breast cancer. Surgical reconstruction is the final step in regaining a sense of complete womanhood, enabling a sense of optimism that both body and self will 'get back to normal'. But what happens when the reconstruction is unsuccessful? What happens to the hope of becoming whole again? When this 'final step' is no longer available women are forced to renegotiate their sense of self without breasts.

The third choice, to reconceptualize her body as normal, feminine and complete without two breasts is utterly absent from breast cancer discourse. To 'do nothing' is not regarded as a decision that is informed and competently made, rather it is a deferral of choice. To continue to allow the mastectomized body to be reproduced as something which is abnormal, unfeminine, desexualized, and incomplete by and for women with breast cancer is to remain silent about other avenues with which women can begin to understand and accept the new materialities of their post-surgical body.

When in hospital recovering from surgery women should not be confronted only with images of restored breasts or have to read or hear that recovery is dependent on their willingness to wear prostheses. Instead, perhaps consumer literature could place more emphasis on readjusting to a body without two breasts and suggest ways to do this; for example, detailing practical tips on altering clothes to remove emphasis from the mastectomy site. In addition, the inclusion of more anecdotes or case studies of women who have not restored their breasts would help normalize the mastectomized body and reduce pressure to wear prostheses.

A woman's acceptance of her changed body must not be dependent on others' acceptance of it. While a woman's view of and feelings about her body cannot be experienced in a social and cultural vacuum, women should be encouraged to look at and touch the mastectomy site, and to experience being one- or no-breasted without feeling they *should* be covering it up. As women come into contact with breast care nurses, medical practitioners and breast cancer volunteers they could be reassured that their body is changed, not abnormal. Being given temporary prostheses immediately after surgery sends a clear message of what is expected. Perhaps removing such devices from sample bags would allow more time for women to readjust to their mastectomized body.

Images of the post-surgical body that openly and honestly portray what a mastectomy looks like should be more publicly available. In doing so the mastectomized body could become normalized and not so potentially challenging to others. Such images could again be included in breast cancer advertising campaigns, and be included in information women are given when diagnosed. In this way the cosmetic result of breast amputation is not unknown to women facing it, and these pictures could be shown to partners, family and friends. This may remove some of the fear women have about revealing their post-surgical body and begin to build their confidence in presenting publicly without two breasts. As noted at the beginning of this book, the public display of a mastectomy has been met with contention from major breast cancer organizations. They claim it is counterproductive to disclose the effects of breast surgery, as it will instill fear and horror in the minds of women. But alternatively it could be argued that images of mastectomies may be productive in encouraging women to attend regular screening of their breasts.

Women who do not wear prostheses should be encouraged to be more visible within breast cancer culture, granting permission to other women to free themselves from the social obligation to 'cover up'. These women should also be at hospital bedsides acting as a literal representation of the normalcy of the post-surgical body and sending a positive message that women do not need breasts to look and feel good about themselves. Seminars and workshops could be developed by breast cancer organizations and advocacy groups which highlight ways women can come to terms with their changed bodies. A workshop for example might focus on building self-confidence, help women rediscover their femininity in ways that do not rely on breasts and remind women that breasts are just one part of a woman's sexuality. A fashion parade that includes women modeling one- or no-breasted would send a clear message that it is okay to look this way, and that it does not mean looking feminine, sexy and 'normal' is unattainable. In these ways women are given the freedom of choice to decide for themselves what breast loss means.

In the conclusion to Barbara's Joss's book *My Left Breast* she states that she is 'complete again' after her reconstruction despite her breast being numb, awaiting her next operation to have a piece of skin from her hip transformed into a nipple, and then waiting to be medically tattooed a few weeks later to colour the nipple and areola. In addition, she states that at the time of the nipple operation other 'adjustments' will be made, such as liposuction on the new and natural breasts to make them look alike. In the postscript to her autobiography she offers tips for transforming one's life. In a list that includes 'knowing myself', 'forgiving myself' and 'accepting love from others', her final 'titbit' is, 'Accepting that I'll never be finished – I'll always be a work-in-progress' (1999: 164).

While one can assume Joss is referring to a more transcendental state of continual self-development, in the context of her narrative it alludes to two things. First, on a physical level she will never be what she was prior to her illness. Even after her breast is reconstructed it is still needing to be 'fixed', and will continue to do so as her body changes and ages over time. In addition, her natural breast will need to be 'adjusted' to maintain symmetry. Secondly, she reveals the 'complete self' that has been restored as false. Instead the self is positioned as something which can never be 'complete', rather it is continually enacted and *done* as different things in different frameworks of meaning. The implication for women who face mastectomy, or who are unhappy with how their post-surgical body looks and feels, is that there are alternatives to having to oblige to a prefigured response to breast loss. In a framework that situates the post-surgical body positively and locates femininity, sexuality and normalcy in things we *do* and *feel* rather than the way we *look*, women can begin to conceptualize a new 'whole' self without two breasts.

Notes

1 An unacceptable body

1. Unpublished interview with Barbara Joss (2003) by the author.
2. Channel 9 (1998), *A Current Affair* (aired on 12/10/98). Interview with Professor Sally Redman.
3. Unpublished interview with Barbara Joss (2003) by the author.
4. *Woman's Day* (1998), 'You have to shock people': Barbara's brave battle, *Woman's Day* 2 November, 1998. Sydney, NSW: ACP Publishing Pty Ltd.
5. Channel 9 (1998), *The Midday Show with Kerri-Anne Kennerley* (aired on 30/11/98). Interview with Barbara Joss.
6. Silverman, David (1987), *Communication and Medical Practice: Social Relations in the Clinic*, London: Sage, p. 14.
7. Mol, Annemarie (1998), Missing links, making links: The performance of some Atheroscleroses, *Differences in Medicine: Unravelling Practices, Techniques, and Bodies*, M. Berg and A. Mol (Eds), London: Duke University Press.
8. Cannon, Sue (1989), Social research in stressful settings: Difficulties for the sociologist studying the treatment of breast cancer, *Sociology of Health and Illness* 11(1): 62–77; Opie, Anne (1992), *There's Nobody There: Community Care of Confused Older People*, Auckland: Oxford University Press.
9. Forbes, J. (1997) The control of breast cancer. The role of tamoxifen, *Seminars in Oncology* 24(1) Supplement 1: S1-5–S1-19.
10. Ibid.
11. Australian Institute of Health and Welfare (2001), *Cancer Survival in Australia 2001* (online), http://www.aihw.gov.au/publications/can/csa01part1/index.html. (Accessed 5/11/02); Peto, R. (1998), Mortality from breast cancer in United Kingdom has decreased suddenly. *British Medical Journal* 317: 476–477; Peto, R. (2000) UK and USA breast cancer deaths down 25% in year 2000 at ages 20–69 years, *Lancet* 355: 1822.
12. Coates, M. and Armstrong, B. (1997), *Cancer in New South Wales: Incidence and Mortality 1994*, Sydney: NSW Cancer Council.
13. Colditz, G. A., Willett, W. C., and Hunter, D. J. (1993), Family history, age, and risk of breast cancer: Prospective data from the Nurses Health Study, *Journal of the American Medical Association* 270: 338.
14. National Health & Medical Research Council (1996), *All about early breast cancer*. Australia: NHMRC.
15. Craft, P., Primrose, J., Lindner, J., and McManus, P. (1997), Surgical management of breast cancer in Australian women in 1993: Analysis of Medicare statistics (online). *Medical Journal of Australia Online*, http://www.mja.com.au. (Accessed 10/9/99); Tulloh, B. and Goldsworthy, M. (1997), Breast cancer management: A rural perspective (online), *Medical Journal of Australia Online*, http://www.mja.com.au (Accessed 10/9/99); Collins, J. (1997), 'Best practice' in surgical management of breast cancer (online), *Medical Journal of Australia Online*, http://www.mja.com.au (Accessed 10/9/99).

16. Craft, P., Primrose, J., Lindner, J. and McManus, P. (1997), Surgical management of breast cancer in Australian women in 1993: Analysis of Medicare statistics (online). *Medical Journal of Australia Online*, http://www.mja.com.au. (Accessed 10/9/99).

17. For an overview, see Wickman, M. (1995), Breast reconstruction – Past achievements, current status and future goals, *Scandinavian Journal of Plastic and Reconstructive Hand Surgery* 29: 81–100.

18. Burcham, Joyce (1997), *Breast Reconstruction: A Review of the Research and Patient and Professional Resources*, NSW: NHMRC National Breast Cancer Centre.

19. See for example: Kasper, Anne S. (1994), A feminist, qualitative methodology: A study of women with breast cancer, *Qualitative Sociology* 17: 263–281; Waxler-Morrison, N., Doll, R., and Hislop, G. (1995), The use of qualitative methods to strengthen psychosocial research on cancer, *Journal of Psychosocial Oncology* 13: 177–191; Rosenbaum, Marcy, and Roos, Gun (2000), Women's experiences of breast cancer. *Breast Cancer: Society Shapes an Epidemic*, A. Kasper and S. Ferguson (Eds), New York: St Martin's Press, pp. 153–182.

20. For examples of review articles of psychosocial literature, see Glanz, Karen, and Lerman, Caryn (1991), Psychosocial impact of breast cancer: A critical review, *Annals of Behavioural Medicine* 14: 204–212; Meyerowitz, B. E. (1980), Psychosocial correlates of breast cancer and its treatments. *Psychological Bulletin* 87: 108–131; Wainstock, J. M. (1991), Breast cancer: Psychosocial consequences for the patient, *Seminars in Oncology Nursing* 7: 207–215.

21. Abrums, Mary (2000), 'Jesus will fix it after a while': Meanings and health, *Social Science and Medicine* 50: 89–105; Wardlow, H. and Curry, R. (1996), 'Sympathy for my body': Breast cancer and mammography at two Atlanta clinics, *Medical Anthropology* 16: 319–340; Kirchgassler, K. (1990), Change and continuity in patient theories of illness: The case of epilepsy, *Social Science and Medicine* 30(12): 1313–1318; Bottorff, J., Johnson, J., Bhagat, R., Grewal, S., Balneaves, L., Clarke, H., and Hilton, A. (1998), Beliefs related to breast health practices: The perceptions of South Asian women living in Canada. *Social Science and Medicine* 47(12): 2075–2085.

22. Kasper, Anne S. (1995), The social construction of breast loss and reconstruction. *Women's Health: Research on Gender, Behaviour and Policy* 1(3): 197–219; Crouch, Mira. and McKenzie, Heather (2000), Social realities of loss and suffering following mastectomy. *Health* 4(2): 196–215; Manderson, Lenore (1999), Gender, normality and the post-surgical body. *Anthropology and Medicine* 6(3): 381–394.

23. Ferguson, Susan J. (2000), Deformities and diseased: The medicalisation of women's breasts. *Breast Cancer: Society Shapes an Epidemic*. A. Kasper and S. Ferguson (Eds), New York: St Martin's Press, pp. 51–86.

24. Crouch, Mira. and McKenzie, Heather (2000), Social realities of loss and suffering following mastectomy. *Health* 4(2): 196–215; Broom, Dorothy (2001), Reading breast cancer: Reflections on a dangerous intersection. *Health* 5(2): 249–268.

25. Crouch, Mira. and McKenzie, Heather (2000), Social realities of loss and suffering following mastectomy. *Health* 4(2): 196–215; Broom, Dorothy. (2001), Reading breast cancer: Reflections on a dangerous intersection. *Health* 5(2): 249–268; Wilkinson, Sue. (2001), Breast cancer: Feminism, representations

and resistance: A commentary on Dorothy Broom's 'Reading Breast Cancer'. *Health* 5(2): 269–278.

26. Wilkinson, Sue (2001), Breast cancer: Feminism, representations and resistance: A commentary on Dorothy Broom's 'Reading Breast Cancer'. *Health* 5(2): 269–278.

27. Young, Iris Marion (1990), *Throwing Like a Girl and Other Essays in Feminist Philosophy and Social Theory*. Bloomington: Indiana University Press.

28. Young, Iris Marion (1990), *Throwing Like a Girl and Other Essays in Feminist Philosophy and Social Theory*. Bloomington: Indiana University Press. p. 153.

29. Butler, Judith (1993), *Bodies That Matter: On the Discursive Limits of 'Sex'*. New York: Routledge, pp. 1–2.

30. Grosz, Elizabeth (1994), *Volatile Bodies: Toward a Corporeal Feminism*. St. Leonards, NSW: Allen & Unwin, p. 23.

31. Lupton, Deborah (1994a), *Medicine as Culture: Illness, Disease and the Body in Western Societies*. London: Sage, p. 17.

32. Ibid., p. 18.

33. Haraway, Donna J. (1997), *Modest_Witness@Second_Millennium.FemaleMan_ Meets_OncoMouse: Feminism and Technoscience*. New York: Routledge.

34. Clarke, Adele and Fujimura, Joan (1992), Chapter One: The right tools for the job. *The Right Tools for the Job*. A. Clarke and J. Fujimura (Eds), Princeton, New Jersey: Princeton University Press, p. 4.

35. Ibid., p. 5.

36. Mol, Annemarie. (1998), Missing links, making links: The performance of some Atheroscleroses. *Differences in Medicine: Unravelling Practices, Techniques, and Bodies*. M. Berg, and A. Mol (Eds), London: Duke University Press; Mol, Annemarie (1999), Ontological politics. A word and some questions. *Actor Network Theory and After*. J. Law and J. Hassard (Eds), Oxford: Blackwell Publishers, pp. 74–89.

37. Butler, Judith (1990), *Gender Trouble: Feminism and the Subversion of Identity*. New York: Routledge.

2 Narratives of the self

1. For detailed reviews of literature on illness narratives see, Bury, Michael (2001), Illness narratives: Fact or fiction? *Sociology of Health and Illness* 23(3): 263–285; Hyden, Lars-Christer (1997), Illness and narrative. *Sociology of Health and Illness* 19(1): 48–69.

2. Hyden, Lars-Christer (1997), Illness and narrative. *Sociology of Health and Illness* 19(1): 48–69, 48.

3. See Kohler Riessman, Catherine (1990), Strategic uses of narrative in the presentation of self and illness: A research note. *Social Science and Medicine* 30(11): 1195–1200; Brody, H. (1987), *Stories of Sickness*. New Haven: Yale University Press; Kleinman, A., Eisenberg, L., and Good, B. (1978), Culture, illness and care: Clinical lessons from anthropologic and cross-cultural research. *Annals of Internal Medicine* 88(2): 251–258; Taylor, C. (1996), *Sources of the Self: The Making of Modern Identity*. Cambridge: Cambridge University Press; Davies, M. (1997), Shattered assumptions: Time and the experience of long-term HIV positivity. *Social Science and Medicine* 44: 561–571.

4. See Little, M., Paul, K., Jordens, C., and Sayers, E.-J. (2000), Vulnerability in the narratives of patients and their carers: Studies of colo-rectal cancer. *Health* 4(4): 499–514; van der Molen, B. (2000), Relating information needs to the cancer experience: Jenny's story – a cancer narrative. *European Journal of Cancer Care* 7(1): 41–47; Mathieson, Cynthia. and Stam, Henderikus (1995), Renegotiating identity: Cancer narratives. *Sociology of Health and Illness* 17(3): 283–306.
5. Crossley, Michele L. (1999), Stories of illness and trauma survival: Liberation or repression? *Social Science and Medicine* 48: 1685.
6. See Abrums, Mary (2000), 'Jesus will fix it after a while': Meanings and health. *Social Science and Medicine* 50: 89–105; Daaleman, T., Kuckelman Cobb, A., and Frey, B. (2001), Spirituality and well-being: An exploratory study of the patient perspective. *Social Science and Medicine* 53: 1503–1511; Radley, Alan and Billig, Michael (1996), Accounts of health and illness: Dilemmas and representations. *Sociology of Health and Illness* 18(2): 220–240.
7. See Sered, Susan and Tabory, Ephraim (1999), 'You are a number, not a human being': Israeli breast cancer patients' experiences with the medical establishment. *Medical Anthropology Quarterly* 13(2): 223–252; Garro, Linda (1994), Narrative representations of chronic illness experience: Cultural models of illness, mind, and body in stories concerning the temporomandibular joint (TMJ). *Social Science and Medicine* 38(6): 775–788; Good, Byron J. (1994), *Medicine, Rationality, and Experience: An Anthropological Perspective.* Cambridge: Cambridge University Press; Gordon, D. and Paci, E. (1997), Disclosure practices and cultural narratives: Understanding concealment and silence around cancer in Tuscany, Italy. *Social Science and Medicine* 44(10): 1433–1452.
8. See Frank, Arthur W. (1993), The rhetoric of self-change: Illness experience as narrative. *The Sociological Quarterly* 34: 39–52; Frank, Arthur W. (1994), Reclaiming an orphan genre: The first-person narrative of illness. *Literature and Medicine* 13: 1–21; Frank, Arthur W. (1995), *The Wounded Storyteller: Body, Illness and Ethics.* Chicago: Chicago University Press; Hyden, Lars-Christer (1997), Illness and narrative. *Sociology of Health and Illness* 19(1): 48–69; Little, M., Jordens, C., Paul, K., Montgomery, K. and Philipson, B. (1998), Liminality: A major category of the experience of cancer illness. *Social Science and Medicine* 47(10): 1485–1494; Williams, Gareth (1984), The genesis of chronic illness: Narrative re-construction. *Sociology of Health and Illness* 6(2): 175–200; Robinson, Ian (1990), Personal narratives, social careers and medical courses: Analysing life trajectories in autobiographies of people with multiple sclerosis. *Social Science and Medicine* 30(11): 1173–1186; Jordens, C., Little, M., Paul, K. and Sayers, E.-J. (2001), Life disruption and generic complexity: A social linguistic analysis of narratives of cancer illness. *Social Science and Medicine* 53: 1227–1236; Ezzy, Douglas (2000), Illness narratives: Time, hope and HIV. *Social Science and Medicine* 50: 605–617; Bury, Michael (2001), Illness narratives: Fact or fiction? *Sociology of Health and Illness* 23(3): 263–285.
9. Frank, Arthur W. (1995), *The Wounded Storyteller: Body, Illness and Ethics.* Chicago: Chicago University Press.
10. Gray, R., Sinding, C. and Fitch, M. (2001), Navigating the social context of metastatic breast cancer: Reflections on a project linking research to drama. *Health* 5(2): 233–248.

11. Saillant, Francine (1990), Discourse, knowledge and experience of cancer: A life story. *Culture, Medicine and Psychiatry* 14: 81–104.
12. Thorne, S. and Murray, C. (2000), Social constructions of breast cancer. *Health Care for Women International* 21: 141–159.
13. Rosenbaum, Marcy and Roos, Gun (2000), Women's experiences of breast cancer. *Breast Cancer: Society Shapes an Epidemic*. A. Kasper and S. Ferguson (Eds), New York: St Martin's Press, p. 177.
14. Saillant, Francine (1990), Discourse, knowledge and experience of cancer: A life story. *Culture, Medicine and Psychiatry* 14: 81–104.
15. Hyden, Lars-Christer (1997), Illness and narrative. *Sociology of Health and Illness* 19(1): 48–69.
16. Babrow, Austin S. and Kline, Kimberly N. (2000), From 'reducing' to 'coping with' uncertainty: Reconceptualizing the central challenge in breast self-exams. *Social Science and Medicine* 51: 1805–1816; Fishman, Jennifer (2000), Assessing breast cancer: Risk, science and environmental activism in an 'at risk' community. *Ideologies of Breast Cancer: Feminist Perspectives*. L. K. Potts (Ed.), London: Macmillan Press Ltd, pp. 181–204; Gifford, Sandra M. (1986), The meaning of lumps: A case study of the ambiguities of risk. *Anthropology and Epidemiology: Interdisciplinary Approaches to the Study of Health and Disease*. C. Janes, R. Stall and S. Gifford (Eds), Boston: D Reidel Publishing Company, pp. 213–246; Hallowell, Nina (2000), Reconstructing the body or reconstructing the woman? Problems of prophylactic mastectomy for hereditary breast cancer risk. *Ideologies of Breast Cancer: Feminist Perspectives*. L. K. Potts (Ed.), London: Macmillan Press Ltd, pp. 153–180; Lock, Margaret (1998), Breast cancer: Reading the omens. *Anthropology Today* 14(4): 7–16; Rees, G., Fry, A. and Cull, A. (2001), A family history of breast cancer: Women's experiences from a theoretical perspective. *Social Science and Medicine* 52: 1433–1440; Robertson, Ann (2001), Biotechnology, political rationality and discourses on health risk. *Health* 5(3): 293–310; Simpson, Christy (2000), Controversies in breast cancer prevention: The discourse of risk. *Ideologies of Breast Cancer: Feminist Perspectives*. L. K. Potts (Ed.), London: Macmillan Press Ltd, pp. 131–152; Yadlon, Susan (1997), Skinny women and good mothers: The rhetoric of risk, control and culpability in the production of knowledge about breast cancer. *Feminist Studies* 23(3): 645–677.
17. Sontag, Susan (1978), *Illness as Metaphor*. New York: Farrar, Straus & Giroux.
18. Ibid.
19. Yadlon, Susan (1997), Skinny women and good mothers: The rhetoric of risk, control and culpability in the production of knowledge about breast cancer. *Feminist Studies* 23(3): 646.
20. Greer, S., Morris, T. and Pettingale, K. W. (1979), Psychological response to breast cancer: Effect on outcome. *The Lancet* ii (13 October): 785–787; Pettingale, K. W., Morris, T., Greer, S. and Haybittle, J. L. (1985), Mental attitudes to cancer: An additional prognostic factor. *The Lancet* (30 March): 750; Dunkel-Shetter, C., Feinstein, L. G., Taylor, S. E. and Falke, R. L. (1992), Patterns of coping with cancer. *Health Psychology* 11: 79–87; Taylor, S. E. (1983), Adjustment to threatening events: A theory of cognitive adaptation. *American Psychologist* 58: 1161–1173; Taylor, S. E. (1989), *Positive Illusions: Creative Self-Deception and the Healthy Mind*. New York: Basic Books; Taylor, S. E. (1990), Health psychology: The science and the field. *American Psychologist* 45: 40–50.

21. Gifford, Sandra M. (1986), The meaning of lumps: A case study of the ambiguities of risk. *Anthropology and Epidemiology: Interdisciplinary Approaches to the Study of Health and Disease*, C. Janes, R. Stall and S. Gifford (Eds), Boston: D Reidel Publishing Company, pp. 213–246.

22. See for example Garrett, Catherine J. (1997), Remaking the self through metaphor: Recovery from anorexia nervosa. *Health* 1:2(October): 139–156; Malson, Helen (1998), *The Thin woman: Feminism, Post-Structuralism and the Social Psychology of Anorexia Nervosa*. London: Routledge.

23. Garrett, Catherine J. (1997), Remaking the self through metaphor: Recovery from anorexia nervosa. *Health* 1:2(October): 145.

24. Bush, Judith (2000), 'It's just part of being a woman': Cervical screening, the body and femininity. *Social Science and Medicine* 50: 429–444; Lupton, Deborah (1994b), Femininity, responsibility, and the technological imperative: Discourses on breast cancer in the Australian press. *International Journal of Health Services* 24(1): 73–89; Saywell, C., Henderson, L. and Beattie, L. (2000), Sexualised illness: The newsworthy body in media representations of breast cancer. *Ideologies of Breast Cancer: Feminist Perspectives*. L. K. Potts (Ed.), London: Macmillan Press Ltd, pp. 37–62.

25. Manderson, Lenore (1999), Gender, normality and the post-surgical body. *Anthropology and Medicine* 6(3): 390.

26. Fife, Betsy L. (1994), The conceptualization of meaning in illness. *Social Science and Medicine* 38(2): 309–316.

27. Freund, P. and McGuire, M. (1999), Chronic illness and disability: The politics of impairment. *Illness, Health and the Social Body*, pp. 154–164; Goffman, Erving (1968), *Stigma: Notes on the Management of Spoiled Identity*. Harmondsworth: Penguin.

28. Mathieson, Cynthia and Stam, Henderikus (1995), Renegotiating identity: Cancer narratives. *Sociology of Health and Illness* 17(3): 283–306; Fosket, Jennifer (2000), Problematising biomedicine: Women's constructions of breast cancer knowledge. *Ideologies of Breast Cancer: Feminist Perspectives*. L. K. Potts (Ed.), London: Macmillan Press Ltd, pp. 15–36.

29. Gwyn, Richard (2003), Processes of refiguration: Shifting identities in cancer narratives, *Discourse, the Body, and Identity*, J. Coupland and R. Gwyn (Eds), New York: Palgrave Macmillan (Houndmills), pp. 209–224.

30. Gifford, Sandra M. (1986), The meaning of lumps: A case study of the ambiguities of risk. *Anthropology and Epidemiology: Interdisciplinary Approaches to the Study of Health and Disease*, C. Janes, R. Stall and S. Gifford (Eds), Boston: D Reidel Publishing Company, p. 238.

31. Hallowell, Nina (2000), Reconstructing the body or reconstructing the woman? Problems of prophylactic mastectomy for hereditary breast cancer risk, *Ideologies of Breast Cancer: Feminist Perspectives*, L. K. Potts (Ed.), London: Macmillan Press Ltd, pp. 153–180.

32. Mechanic, D. (1968), *Medical Sociology*. New York: Free Press; Murcott, A. (1981), On the typification of bad patients, *Medical Work, Realities and Routines*, P. Atkinson and C. Heath (Eds), London: Gower, pp. 128–140; Bloor, M. and Horobin, G. (1975), Conflict and conflict resolution in doctor-patient interactions, *A Sociology of Medical Practice*, C. Cox and A. Mead (Eds), London: Macmillan.

33. Reaby, Linda L. (1996), *Post-Mastectomy Self-Perceptions, Attitudes and Breast Restoration Decision-Making*, Canberra: University of Canberra; Reaby, Linda L.

(1998a), Breast restoration decision making: Enhancing the process, *Cancer Nursing* 21(3): 196–204; Reaby, Linda L. (1998b), Reasons why women who have mastectomy decide to have or not to have breast reconstruction, *Plastic and Reconstructive Surgery* 101(7): 1810–1818; Reaby, Linda L. (1999), Breast restoration decision making, *Plastic Surgical Nursing* 19(1): 22–30; Reaby, Linda L., Hort, Linda, K. and Vandervord, John (1994), Body image, self-concept and self-esteem in women who had a mastectomy and either wore an external breast prosthesis or had breast reconstruction and women who had not experienced mastectomy, *Health Care for Women International* 15: 361–375; Reaby, Linda L. and Hort, Linda K. (1995), Post-mastectomy attitudes in women who wear external breast prostheses compared to those who have undergone breast reconstructions. *Journal of Behavioural Medicine* 18(1): 55–67; Price, B. (1992), Living with altered body image: The cancer experience, *British Journal of Nursing* 1(3): 641–645; Handel, N., Silverstein, M., Waisman, E. and Waisman, J. (1990), Reasons why mastectomy patients do not have breast reconstruction, *Plastic and Reconstructive Surgery* 86(6): 1118–1122; Mock, V. (1993), Body image in women treated for breast cancer, *Nursing Research* 42(30): 153–157.

3 Pink advocacy: Camaraderie, competition and the making of a breast cancer career

1. Orbach, S. (1988), *Fat is a Feminist Issue*, London: Arrow Books; Bartky, S. (1990), *Femininity and Domination: Studies in the Phenomenology of Oppression*, New York: Routledge; Smith, D. E. (1990), *Texts, Facts and Femininity: Exploring the Relations of Ruling*. London: Routledge; Young, Iris Marion (1990), *Throwing Like a Girl and Other Essays in Feminist Philosophy and Social Theory*, Bloomington: Indiana University Press; Ussher, Jane (1992), Reproductive rhetoric and the blaming of the body, *The Psychology of Women's Health and Health Care*, P. Nicholson and J. Ussher (Eds), London: Macmillan Press Ltd, pp. 31–61.
2. Batt, Sharon (1994), *Patient No More: The Politics of Breast Cancer*, Melbourne: Spinifex.
3. Klawiter, Maren (2000), Racing for the cure, walking women and toxic touring: Mapping cultures of action within the Bay Area terrain of breast cancer, *Ideologies of Breast Cancer: Feminist Perspectives*, L. K. Potts (Ed.), London: Macmillan Press Ltd, pp. 63–97; Kaufert, Patricia A. (1998), Women, resistance, and the breast cancer movement. *Pragmatic Women and Body Politics*. M. Lock and P. Kaufert (Eds), Cambridge: Cambridge University Press, pp. 287–309; Montini, T. (1996), Gender and emotion in the advocacy of breast cancer informed consent legislation. *Gender and Society* 10: 9–23; Taylor, V. and Van Willigen, M. (1996), Women's self help and the reconstruction of gender: The postpartum support and breast cancer movements. *Mobilization: An International Journal* 1: 123–143; Anglin, Mary K. (1997), Working from the inside out: Implications of breast cancer activism for biomedical policies and practices. *Social Science and Medicine* 44(9): 1403–1415. Brenner, Barbara 2000, Sister Support: Women create a breast cancer movement. *Breast Cancer: Society Shapes an epidemic*, A. Kasper and S. Ferguson (Eds), New York: St Martin's Press, pp. 325–354.

4. Montini, T. (1996), Gender and emotion in the advocacy of breast cancer informed consent legislation. *Gender and Society* 10: 9–23; Taylor, V. and Van Willigen, M. (1996), Women's self help and the reconstruction of gender: The postpartum support and breast cancer movements. *Mobilization: An International Journal* 1: 123–143.

5. Anglin, Mary K. (1997), Working from the inside out: Implications of breast cancer activism for biomedical policies and practices. *Social Science and Medicine* 44(9): 1403–1415; Taylor, V. and Van Willigen, M. (1996), Women's self help and the reconstruction of gender: The postpartum support and breast cancer movements, *Mobilization: An International Journal* 1: 123–143.

6. Anglin, Mary K. (1997), Working from the inside out: Implications of breast cancer activism for biomedical policies and practices. *Social Science and Medicine* 44(9): 1403–1415.

7. American Cancer Society, www.cancer.org. In Australia state-based Cancer Councils were established in South Australia (1928), Victoria (1936), NSW (1955), Western Australia (1955), Queensland (1961), and the ACT (1976).

8. Stevens, Joyce (1995), *Healing Women: A History of Leichhardt Women's Community Health Centre*, Leichhardt, NSW: First Ten Years History Project; Broom, Dorothy (1991), *Damned If We Do: Contradictions in Women's Health Care*, Sydney: Allen & Unwin.

9. NSW, QLD and SA – 1975; WA – 1977; ACT – 1981.

10. The Reach to Recovery website is found at *International Union Against Cancer*, www.uicc.org.

11. For example, Bosom Buddies, Alice Springs, NT Breast Cancer Voice, BC Support Group, Mt Isa, B 'r'est Friends, Bundaberg, Fenceliners, Qld, Action for Breast Cancer SA, Caring Cancer Support group, Port Lincoln, BC foundation of WA, The Devonport BC and Lymphodema Support Group, Forget-Me-Nots BCSG, Vic, Daffodils BCSG, Vic, Power Pals Breast cancer support group, NSW, Dragons Abreast, ACT, Qld, Vic, NSW, WA, to name but a few . . .

12. Australia. Dept of Community Services and Health (1989), *National Women's Health Policy: Advancing Women's Health in Australia*. Canberra: Australian Government Publishing Service: 36.

13. Number of groups from each state in 2002: NSW – 29, VIC – 29, ACT – 4, TAS – 2, SA – 15, WA – 2, NT – 3, QLD – 13).

14. See Broom, Dorothy (1991), *Damned If We Do: Contradictions in Women's Health Care*. Sydney: Allen & Unwin.

15. For example, the Warrior Women art exhibition, a collection of art by women exploring their experiences of breast cancer. This exhibition toured around Australia in 2002. See Royal Women's Hospital (2002), Women's art @whic (online), *Wellwomen's Website*, http://www.rwh.org.au/wellwomens/whic.cfm?doc_id=2446 (Accessed 10/9/03).

16. Yadlon, Susan (1997), Skinny women and good mothers: The rhetoric of risk, control and culpability in the production of knowledge about breast cancer. *Feminist Studies* 23(3): 645–677.

17. Saywell, C., Henderson, L. and Beattie, L. (2000), Sexualised illness: The newsworthy body in media representations of breast cancer, *Ideologies of Breast Cancer: Feminist Perspectives*. L. K. Potts (Ed.), London: Macmillan Press Ltd, pp. 37–62; Lupton, Deborah (1994b), Femininity, responsibility, and the

technological imperative: Discourses on breast cancer in the Australian press. *International Journal of Health Services* 24(1): 73–89.

18. Lupton, Deborah (1994b), Femininity, responsibility, and the technological imperative: Discourses on breast cancer in the Australian press. *International Journal of Health Services* 24(1): 73–89; Lantz, P. and Booth, K. (1998), The social construction of the breast cancer epidemic. *Social Science and Medicine* 46(7): 907–918; McKay, S. and Bonner, F. (1999), Telling stories: Breast cancer pathographies in Australian women's magazines. *Women's Studies International Forum* 22(5): 563–571.
19. Images can be found at http://hosted.aware.easynet.co.uk/jospence/jo1.htm.
20. Cartwright, Lisa (1998), Community and the public body in breast cancer media activism. *Cultural Studies* 12(2): 123.
21. Gray, R., Sinding, C. and Fitch, M. (2001), Navigating the social context of metastatic breast cancer: Reflections on a project linking research to drama. *Health* 5(2): 233–248.
22. Lorde, Audre (1980), The Cancer Journals, reprinted in *The Audre Lorde* compendium: Essays, speeches and journals (1996), London: Pandora, p. 59.
23. Klawiter, Maren (2000), Racing for the cure, walking women and toxic touring: Mapping cultures of action within the Bay Area terrain of breast cancer. *Ideologies of Breast Cancer: Feminist Perspectives.* L. K. Potts (Ed.), London: Macmillan Press Ltd, p. 89.
24. Davis, Kathy (1994), *Reshaping the Female Body: The Dilemmas of Cosmetic Surgery*, London: Routledge.

4 Practices and prostheses

1. Amoena-Coloplast (1999), *Luxa Contact: Confidence that Sticks With You.* Marietta, Georgia: Coloplast Corporation, p. 1.
2. Amoena-Coloplast Corporation (2003b), *Amoena-Coloplast Corporation Website*, (online). http://www.coloplast.com (Accessed 5/7/03).
3. Breast Cancer Forum (2002), How to make a millet prosthesis (online), *Breast Cancer Forum Website*, http://www.bcforum.org. (Accessed 15/5/02).
4. About Breast Cancer (2002), *How to Make a Spare Seed Prosthesis* (online), http://breastcancer.about.com/c/ht/00/07/How_Spare_Seed_Prosthesis 0962934723.htm. (Accessed 13/5/02).
5. Kasper, Anne S. (1995), The social construction of breast loss and reconstruction. *Women's Health: Research on Gender, Behaviour and Policy* 1(3): 205.
6. Turner, Bryan S. (1992), *Regulating Bodies: Essays in Medical Sociology*. USA: Routledge, p. 15.
7. Hardey, Michael (1999), Doctor in the house: The Internet as a source of lay health knowledge and the challenge to expertise. *Sociology of Health and Illness* 21(6): 820–835; Sharf, Barbara F. (1997), Communicating breast cancer on-line: Support and empowerment on the Internet. *Women & Health* 26(1): 65–84.
8. See for example: Australian Cancer Society (1991), *Moving Ahead*; Australian Cancer Society (2000), *After Breast Cancer Surgery: Looking Ahead*; Cancer Council NSW (1998), *Understanding Sexuality and Cancer*; NHMRC (1995), *A Consumer's Guide: Early Breast Cancer*; NHMRC (1996), *All About Early Breast*

Cancer; Queensland Cancer Fund (2000), *A Guide for the Partners of Women with Breast Cancer: How to Help*; Cancer Council NSW (2002), *Emotions and Cancer: A Guide for People With Cancer, Their Families and Friends.*

9. Australian Cancer Society (2000), *After Breast Cancer Surgery: Looking Ahead.* Sydney: Australian Cancer Society.
10. National Health & Medical Research Council (1996), *All About Early Breast Cancer.* Australia: NHMRC, p. 60.
11. Cancer Council NSW (2002), *Emotions and Cancer: A Guide for People With Cancer, Their Families and Friends.* NSW: Cancer Council NSW, pp. 23–24.
12. Calvary Public/Private Hospital (2002), *Breast Care Package*, Canberra: Calvary Public and Private Hospitals Inc. p. 18.
13. Anita-Care (2001), *Tender Body Care After Breast Surgery.* Austria: Anita – Unique Body Wear: 1.
14. Haraway, Donna J. (1997), *Modest_Witness@Second_Millennium.FemaleMan_ Meets_OncoMouse: Feminism and Technoscience.* New York: Routledge.
15. Amoena-Coloplast Corporation (2003b), *Amoena-Coloplast Corporation website*, (online). http://www.coloplast.com (Accessed 5/7/03).
16. Amoena-Coloplast, 2001b, *What Every Woman Who Has Breast Cancer Should Know.* Qld, Australia: Coloplast Pty Ltd. p. 1.
17. Anita-Care (2001), *Tender Body Care After Breast Surgery.* Austria: Anita – Unique Body Wear, p. 2.
18. Ibid., p. 3.
19. Amoena-Coloplast (2001b), *What Every Woman Who Has Had Breast Cancer Should Know.* Qld, Australia: Coloplast Pty Ltd.
20. Amoena-Coloplast (2001a), *Balancia: Creating the Perfect Balance.* Qld, Australia: Coloplast Pty Ltd, p. 2.
21. Ibid., p. 3.
22. Ibid.
23. Kiefer, Carol (2001). Presenting all the choices: Teaching women about breast prosthetics (online). *Medscape Ob/Gyn & Women's Health* 6(5), http://www.medscape.com/viewarticle/408954. (Accessed 4/9/02).
24. Amoena-Coloplast (2001a), *Balancia: Creating the Perfect Balance.* Qld, Australia: Coloplast Pty Ltd, p. 3.
25. Amoena-Coloplast (1999), *Luxa Contact: Confidence That Sticks With You.* Marietta, Georgia: Coloplast Corporation, p. 2.
26. Amoena-Coloplast (2000), *Helping You Stay in Top Form After Breast Surgery.* Qld, Australia: Coloplast Pty Ltd, p. 2.
27. Amoena-Coloplast (1999), *Luxa Contact: Confidence that Sticks With You.* Marietta, Georgia: Coloplast Corporation, p. 4.
28. Amoena-Coloplast Corporation (2003b), *Amoena-Coloplast Corporation Website*, (online). http://www.coloplast.com (Accessed 5/7/03).

5   Breast reconstruction

1. The 'silicone scare' of the 1990s that linked silicone gel to autoimmune disease prompted many thousands of women to go back under the knife and have their implants removed. According to Healy (1998) this dramatic reaction was based on unfounded claims, as the FDA, who placed the moratorium on

silicone breast implants, found no evidence to support removing the implants from the market. Women were left believing there was a 'time bomb' in their bodies and rushed to have them removed (Healy, 1998: 639). This chaos persisted despite the results from well over 15 major clinical trials worldwide finding no scientific basis linking the implants to systemic autoimmune disease (Coope and Dennison, 1998; Healy, 1998). In contrast to this, other studies have pointed out the undeniable complications women have had with implants, and the problems consumers have had in getting these recognised (Lowrey, 1990). A complete history of the controversy surrounding silicone implants can be found in Nora Jacobson (2000), *Cleavage: Technology, Controversy, and the Ironies of the Man-Made Breast*. New Jersey: Rutgers University Press.

2. Wijsbek, H. (2000), The pursuit of beauty: The enforcement of aesthetics or a freely adopted lifestyle? *Journal of Medical Ethics* 26(6): 454.

3. Pauly Morgan, Kathryn (1991), Women and the knife: Cosmetic surgery and the colonisation of women's bodies. *Hypatia* 6(3): 47.

4. Davis, Kathy (1994), *Reshaping the Female Body: The Dilemmas of Cosmetic Surgery*. London: Routledge, p. 163.

5. Williams, Simon J. (1997), Modern medicine and the 'uncertain body': From corporeality to hyperreality? *Social Science and Medicine* 45(7): 1043.

6. Medicare forms the basis of Australia's public health care system aiming to give all Australians access to free or low-cost medical, optometrical and hospital care while individuals are free to choose private health services and in special circumstances allied health services. Medicare provides access to: free treatment as a public (Medicare) patient in a public hospital; free or subsidised treatment by practitioners such as doctors, including specialists, participating optometrists or dentists (specified services only). For more information see the Australian Government Health Insurance Commission website: http://www.hic.gov.au/yourhealth/our_services/medicare/about_medicare/what_is_mc.htm.

7. Glanz, Karen. and Lerman, Caryn (1991), Psychosocial impact of breast cancer: A critical review. *Annals of Behavioural Medicine* 14: 204–212; Meyerowitz, B. E. (1980), Psychosocial correlates of breast cancer and its treatments. *Psychological Bulletin* 87: 108–131; Wainstock, J. M. (1991), Breast cancer: Psychosocial consequences for the patient, *Seminars in Oncology Nursing* 7: 207–215.

8. Handel, N., Silverstein, M., Waisman, E. and Waisman, J. (1990), Reasons why mastectomy patients do not have breast reconstruction, *Plastic and Reconstructive Surgery* 86(6): 1118–1122; Reaby, Linda L. (1998b), Reasons why women who have mastectomy decide to have or not to have breast reconstruction, *Plastic and Reconstructive Surgery* 101(7): 1810–1818; Reaby, Linda L., Hort, Linda, K. and Vandervord, John (1994), Body image, self-concept, and self-esteem in women who had a mastectomy and either wore an external breast prosthesis or had breast reconstruction and women who had not experienced mastectomy. *Health Care for Women International* 15: 361–375; Mock, V. (1993), Body image in women treated for breast cancer. *Nursing Research* 42(30): 153–157; Pierce, P. F. (1993), Deciding on breast cancer treatment: A description of decision-making behaviour. *Nursing Research* 42(22): 22–28; Price, B. (1992), Living with altered body image: The cancer experience. *British Journal of Nursing* 1(3): 641–645.

162   *Notes*

9. Rowland, J., Dioso, J., Holland, J., Chaglassian, T. and Kinne, D. (1995), Breast reconstruction after mastectomy: Who seeks it, who refuses? *Plastic and Reconstructive Surgery* 95(5): 812–822.
10. Shain, W., Wellisch, D., Pasnau, R. and Landsverk, J. (1985), The sooner the better: A study of psychological factors in undergoing immediate versus delayed breast reconstruction. *American Journal of Psychiatry* 142(40); Franchelli, S., Stella Leone, M., Berrino, P., Passarelli, B., Capelli, M., Baracco, G., Alberisio, A., Morasso, G. and Luigi Santi, P. (1995), Psychological evaluation of patients undergoing breast reconstruction using two different methods: Autologous tissues versus prostheses. *Plastic and Reconstructive Surgery* 95(7): 1213–1220.
11. Scanlon, Edward F. (1991), The role of reconstruction in breast cancer. *Cancer* 68(5): 1144–1147; Wickman, M. (1995), Breast reconstruction – Past achievements, current status and future goals. *Scandinavian Journal of Plastic and Reconstructive Hand Surgery* 29: 81–100; Pennington, David (1999), Reconstructions: Expert opinions in B. Joss (Ed.), *My Left Breast: How Breast Cancer Transformed My Life*, Sydney: Joss & Co., pp. 127–134; The Australian Society of Plastic Surgeons (2001), Breast reconstruction after mastectomy (online), *ASPS Website*, http://www.plasticsurgery.org.au/public/aspsframe.asp. (Accessed 5/7/03).
12. Leopold, Ellen (1999), *A Darker Ribbon: Breast Cancer, Women, and Their Doctors in the Twentieth Century*. Boston: Beacon Press; Lerner, Baron (2000), Inventing a curable disease: Historical perspectives on breast cancer. *Breast Cancer: Society Shapes an Epidemic*. A. Kasper and S. Ferguson (Eds) New York: St Martin's Press, pp. 25–50.
13. Doyal, Lesley (1991), The politics of women and surgery: Keynote address. *Proceedings of the Women and Surgery Conference 1990*. R. Moore (Ed.), Melbourne: Healthsharing Women, pp. 59–62.
14. Davis, Kathy (1998), Pygmalions in plastic surgery. *Health* 2(1): 24.
15. Ferguson, Susan J. (2000), Deformities and diseased: The medicalisation of women's breasts. *Breast Cancer: Society Shapes an Epidemic*. A. Kasper and S. Ferguson (Eds), New York: St Martin's Press, p. 54.
16. Franklin, Sarah (1997), *Embodied Progress: A Cultural Account of Assisted Conception*. London: Routledge.

6   Conclusions

1. Fosket, Jennifer (2000), Problematising biomedicine: Women's constructions of breast cancer knowledge. *Ideologies of Breast Cancer: Feminist Perspectives*. L. K. Potts (Ed.), London: Macmillan Press Ltd, pp. 15–36.
2. Rosenbaum, Marcy and Roos, Gun (2000), Women's experiences of breast cancer. *Breast Cancer: Society Shapes an Epidemic*. A. Kasper and S. Ferguson (Eds) New York: St Martin's Press, pp. 153–182.
3. Thorne, S. and Murray, C. (2000), Social constructions of breast cancer. *Health Care for Women International* 21: 141–159.
4. Gifford, Sandra M. (1986), The meaning of lumps: A case study of the ambiguities of risk. *Anthropology and Epidemiology: Interdisciplinary Approaches to the Study of Health and Disease*. C. Janes, R. Stall and S. Gifford (Eds), Boston: D Reidel Publishing Company. pp. 213–246; Mathieson, Cynthia and Stam,

Henderikus (1995), Renegotiating identity: Cancer narratives. *Sociology of Health and Illness* 17(3): 283–306; Parsons, Talcott (1951), *The Social System.* London: Routledge & Kegan Paul.

5. Garrett, Catherine J. (1997), Remaking the self through metaphor: Recovery from anorexia nervosa. *Health* 1(2) (October): 139–156; Malson, Helen (1998), The thin woman: Feminism, post-structuralism and the social psychology of anorexia nervosa. London: Routledge.

6. Manderson, Lenore (1999), Gender, normality and the post-surgical body. *Anthropology and Medicine* 6(3): 381–394.

Bibliography

About Breast Cancer (2002), *How to Make a Spare Seed Prosthesis* (online), http://breast-cancer.about.com/c/ht/00/07/How_Spare_Seed_Prosthesis0962934723.htm. (Accessed 13/5/02).

Abrums, Mary (2000), 'Jesus will fix it after a while': Meanings and health. *Social Science and Medicine* 50: 89–105.

Amoena-Coloplast (1992), *How a Breast Form is Born* (film). USA: Amoena-Coloplast Corporation.

—— (1999), *Luxa Contact: Confidence That Sticks With You*. Marietta, Georgia: Coloplast Corporation.

—— (2000), *Helping You Stay in Top Form after Breast Surgery*. Qld, Australia: Coloplast Pty Ltd.

—— (2001a), *Balancia: Creating the Perfect Balance*. Qld, Australia: Coloplast Pty Ltd.

—— (2001b), *What Every Woman Who Has Had Breast Cancer Should Know*. Qld, Australia: Coloplast Pty Ltd.

Amoena-Coloplast Corporation (2003a), Amoena-Coloplast products (online), *Amoena-Coloplast Corporation website*, http://www.coloplast.com/products. (Accessed 5/7/03).

—— (2003b), *Amoena-Coloplast Corporation website* (online), http://www.colo-plast.com. (Accessed 5/7/03).

Anglin, Mary K. (1997), Working from the inside out: Implications of breast cancer activism for biomedical policies and practices. *Social Science and Medicine* 44(9): 1403–1415.

Anita-Care (2001), *Tender Body Care After Breast Surgery*. Austria: Anita – Unique Body Wear.

Antoni, M. H., Lehman, J. M., Kilbourn, K. M., Boyers, A. E., Culver, J. L., Alferi, S. M., Yount, S. E., McGregor, B. A., Arena, P. L., Harris, S. D., Price, A. A. and Carver, C. S. (2001), Cognitive-behavioural stress management intervention decreases the prevalence of depression and enhances benefit finding among women under treatment for early-stage breast cancer. *Health Psychology* 20(1): 20–32, January.

Ashing-Giwa, K. T., Padilla, G., Tejero, J., Kraemer, J., Wright, K., Coscarelli, A., Clayton, S., Williams, I. and Hills, D. (2004), Understanding the breast cancer experience of women: A qualitative study of African American, Asian American, Latina and Caucasian cancer survivors. *Psycho-Oncology* 13(6): 408–428 June.

Australia Dept of Community Services and Health (1989), National women's health policy: Advancing women's health in Australia. Canberra: Australian Government Publishing Service.

Australian Cancer Society (1991), *Moving Ahead*. Sydney: Australian Cancer Society.

—— (2000), *After Breast Cancer Surgery: Looking Ahead*. Sydney: Australian Cancer Society.

Australian Institute of Health and Welfare (1999), *Breast Cancer in Australian Women 1982–1996* (online), http://www.aihw.gov.au/publications/health/bcaw82–96/index.html (Accessed 8/9/03).

—— (2001), *Cancer Survival in Australia 2001* (online), http://www.aihw.gov.au/publications/can/csa01part1/index.html. (Accessed 5/11/02).

Avis, N. E., Crawford, S. and Manuel, J. (2004), Psychosocial problems among younger women with breast cancer. *Psycho-Oncology* 13(5): 295–308 May.

Babrow, Austin, S. and Kline, Kimberly, N. (2000), From 'reducing' to 'coping with' uncertainty: Reconceptualizing the central challenge in breast self-exams. *Social Science and Medicine* 51: 1805–1816.

Bartky, S. (1990), *Femininity and Domination: Studies in the Phenomenology of Oppression*. New York: Routledge.

Batt, Sharon (1994), *Patient No More: The Politics of Breast Cancer*. Melbourne: Spinifex.

Berg, Bruce, L. (1998), *Qualitative Research Methods for the Social Sciences*. USA: Allyn and Bacon.

Bloom, J. R. and Spiegel, D. (1984), The relationship of 2 dimensions of social support to the psychological well-being and social functioning of women with advanced breast-cancer. *Social Science & Medicine* 19(8): 831–837.

Bloom, J., Stewart, S., Johnston, M., Banks, P. and Fobair, P. (2001), Sources of support and the physical and mental well-being of young women with breast cancer. *Social Science and Medicine* 53: 1513–1524.

Bloor, M. and Horobin, G. (1975), Conflict and conflict resolution in doctor-patient interactions. *A Sociology of Medical Practice*, C. Cox and A. Mead (Eds), London: Macmillan.

Bold, R. J. (2002), Surgical management of breast cancer: Today and tomorrow. *Cancer Biotherapy and Radiopharmaceuticals* 17 (1): 1–9 February.

Bosom Buddies (2003a), Who are Bosom Buddies? (online), *Bosom Buddies website*, http://www.bosombuddies.com.au/identity.htm. (Accessed 15/3/03).

—— (2003b), Field of women photograph (online), *Bosom Buddies website*, http://www.bosombuddies.com.au. (Accessed 15/3/03).

Bottorff, J., Johnson, J., Bhagat, R., Grewal, S., Balneaves, L., Clarke, H. and Hilton, A. (1998), Beliefs related to breast health practices: The perceptions of South Asian women living in Canada. *Social Science and Medicine* 47(12): 2075–2085.

Breast Cancer Action Group (2004), *BCAG Newsletter*. Breast Cancer Action Group, Victoria. No. 56, June.

Breast Cancer Forum (2002), How to make a millet prosthesis (online), *Breast Cancer Forum website*, http://www.bcforum.org. (Accessed 15/5/02).

Breast Cancer Network Australia (2001), History of the BCNA (online), *BCNA website*, http://www.bcna.org.au/about_us/about_us_index.htm (Accessed 13/5/02).

—— (2003a), Logo of the BCNA (online), *BCNA website*, http://www.bcna.com.au. (Accessed 13/5/02).

—— (2003b), A seat the table program (online), *BCNA website*, http://www.bcna.org.au/projects_resources/projects_index.htm. (Accessed 17/7/03).

Brenner, Barbara (2000), Sister support: Women create a breast cancer movement. *Breast Cancer: Society Shapes An Epidemic*, A. Kasper and S. Ferguson (Eds). New York: St Martin's Press, 325–354.

Brody, H. (1987), *Stories of Sickness*. New Haven: Yale University Press.

Broom, Dorothy (1991), *Damned If We Do: Contradictions in Women's Health Care*. Sydney: Allen & Unwin.

—— (2001), Reading breast cancer: Reflections on a dangerous intersection. *Health* 5(2): 249–268.

Burcham, Joyce (1997), *Breast Reconstruction: A Review of the Research and Patient and Professional Resources*. NSW: NHMRC National Breast Cancer Centre.

Bury, Michael (2001), Illness narratives: Fact or fiction? *Sociology of Health and Illness* 23(3): 263–285.

Bush, Judith (2000), 'It's just part of being a woman': Cervical screening, the body and femininity. *Social Science and Medicine* 50: 429–444.

Butler, Judith (1990), *Gender Trouble: Feminism and the Subversion of Identity*. New York: Routledge.

—— (1993), *Bodies that Matter: On the Discursive Limits of 'Sex'*. New York: Routledge.

Calvary Public/Private Hospital (2002), *Breast Care Package*. Canberra: Calvary Public and Private Hospitals Inc.

Cancer Council NSW (1998), *Understanding Sexuality and Cancer*. Sydney, Australia: NSW Cancer Council.

—— (2002), *Emotions and Cancer: A Guide for People with Cancer, Their Families and Friends*. NSW: Cancer Council NSW.

Cancer Council WA (2002), *Fact Sheet*. Cancer Council WA.

Cannon, Sue (1989), Social research in stressful settings: Difficulties for the sociologist studying the treatment of breast cancer. *Sociology of Health and Illness* 11(1): 62–77.

Cartwright, Lisa (1998), Community and the public body in breast cancer media activism. *Cultural Studies* 12(2): 117–138.

Channel 9 (1998), *A Current Affair* (aired on 12/10/98). Interview with Professor Sally Redman.

—— (1998), *The Midday Show with Kerri-Anne Kennerley* (aired on 30/11/98). Interview with Barbara Joss.

Charles, C., Gafni, A. and Whelan, T. (1999), Decision-making in the physician-patient encounter: Revisiting the shared treatment decision-making model. *Social Science and Medicine* 49: 651–661.

Clarke, Adele and Fujimura, Joan (1992), Chapter One: The right tools for the job. *The Right Tools for the Job*, A. Clarke and J. Fujimura (Eds). Princeton, New Jersey: Princeton University Press.

Coates, M. and Armstrong, B. (1997), *Cancer in New South Wales: Incidence and Mortality 1994*. Sydney: NSW Cancer Council.

Cody, H. S. (2002), Current surgical management of breast cancer. *Current Opinion in Obstetrics & Gynaecology* 14(1): 45–52 February.

Colditz, G. A., Willett, W. C. and Hunter, D. J. (1993), Family history, age, and risk of breast cancer: Prospective data from the Nurses Health Study. *Journal of the American Medical Association* 270: 338.

Collins, J. (1997), 'Best practice' in surgical management of breast cancer (online), *Medical Journal of Australia Online*, http://www.mja.com.au. (Accessed 10/9/99).

Coope, C. and Dennison, E. (1998), Editorial: Do silicone breast implants cause connective tissue disease? *British Medical Journal* 316: 403–404.

Cosgrove, Lisa (2000), Crying out loud: Understanding women's emotional distress as both lived experience and social construction. *Feminism and Psychology* 10(2): 247–267.

Cotterill, Pamela (1992), Interviewing women: Issues of friendship, vulnerability, and power. *Women's Studies International Forum* 15(5/6): 593–606.

Craft, P., Primrose, J., Lindner, J. and McManus, P. (1997), Surgical management of breast cancer in Australian women in 1993: Analysis of Medicare statistics (online), *Medical Journal of Australia Online*, http://www.mja.com.au. (Accessed 10/9/99).

Craigie, J. E., Allen, R. J. and DellaCroce, F. J. (2003), Autogenous breast reconstruction with the deep inferior epigastric perforator flap. *Clinics in Plastic Surgery* 30(3): 359.

Crompvoets, Samantha (2001), Interview with Dr David Pennington. Unpublished.

—— (2003), Interview with Barbara Joss. Unpublished.

Crossley, Michele L. (1999), Stories of illness and trauma survival: Liberation or repression? *Social Science and Medicine* 48: 1685–1695.

Crouch, Mira. and McKenzie, Heather (2000), Social realities of loss and suffering following mastectomy. *Health* 4(2): 196–215.

Daaleman, T., Kuckelman Cobb, A. and Frey, B. (2001), Spirituality and well-being: An exploratory study of the patient perspective. *Social Science and Medicine* 53: 1503–1511.

Davies, M. (1997), Shattered assumptions: Time and the experience of long-term HIV positivity. *Social Science and Medicine* 44: 561–571.

Davis, Kathy (1991), Remaking the She-Devil: A critical look at feminist approaches to beauty. *Hypatia* 6: 21–43.

—— (1994), *Reshaping the Female Body: The Dilemmas of Cosmetic Surgery*. London: Routledge.

—— (1998), Pygmalions in plastic surgery. *Health* 2(1): 23–40.

Deadman, J., Leinster, S., Owens, R., Dewey, M. and Slade, P. (2001), Taking responsibility for cancer treatment. *Social Science and Medicine* 53: 669–677.

Doyal, Lesley (1991), The politics of women and surgery: Keynote address. *Proceedings of the Women and Surgery Conference 1990*, R. Moore (Ed.). Melbourne: Healthsharing Women, pp. 59–62.

Dunkel-Shetter, C., Feinstein, L. G., Taylor, S. E. and Falke, R. L. (1992), Patterns of coping with cancer. *Health Psychology* 11: 79–87.

Ehrenreich, Barbara (2001), Welcome to Cancerland. *Harper's Magazine*, November: 43–53.

Entwistle, V., Skea, Z. and O'Donnell, M. (2001), Decisions about treatment: Interpretations of two measures of control by women having a hysterectomy. *Social Science and Medicine* 53: 721–732.

Ezzy, Douglas (2000), Illness narratives: Time, hope and HIV. *Social Science and Medicine* 50: 605–617.

Ferguson, Susan J. (2000), Deformities and diseased: The medicalisation of women's breasts. *Breast Cancer: Society Shapes an Epidemic*, A. Kasper and S. Ferguson (Eds). New York: St Martin's Press, pp. 51–86.

Ferguson, Susan J. and Kasper, Anne S. (2000), Introduction – Living with breast cancer. *Breast Cancer: Society Shapes an Epidemic*, A. Kasper and S. Ferguson (Eds). New York: St Martin's Press, pp. 1–22.

Fife, Betsy L. (1994), The conceptualization of meaning in illness. *Social Science and Medicine* 38(2): 309–316.

Fishman, Jennifer (2000), Assessing breast cancer: Risk, science and environmental activism in an 'at risk' community. *Ideologies of Breast Cancer: Feminist Perspectives*, L. K. Potts (Ed.), London: Macmillan Press Ltd, pp. 181–204.

Forbes, J. (1997), The control of breast cancer. The role of tamoxifen. *Seminars in Oncology* 24(1), Supplement 1: S1-5–S1-19.

Fosket, Jennifer (2000), Problematising biomedicine: Women's constructions of breast cancer knowledge. *Ideologies of Breast Cancer: Feminist Perspectives*, L. K. Potts (Ed.). London: Macmillan Press Ltd, pp. 15–36.

Fosket, Jennifer, Karran, Angela and LaFia, Christine (2000), Breast cancer in popular women's magazines from 1913 to 1996. *Breast Cancer: Society Shapes an Epidemic*, A. Kasper and S. Ferguson (Eds). New York: St Martin's Press. pp. 303–324.

Franchelli, S., Stella Leone, M., Berrino, P., Passarelli, B., Capelli, M., Baracco, G., Alberisio, A., Morasso, G. and Luigi Santi, P. (1995), Psychological evaluation of patients undergoing breast reconstruction using two different methods: Autologous tissues versus prostheses. *Plastic and Reconstructive Surgery* 95(7): 1213–1220.

Frank, Arthur W. (1993), The rhetoric of self-change: Illness experience as narrative. *The Sociological Quarterly* 34: 39–52.

—— (1994), Reclaiming an orphan genre: The first-person narrative of illness. *Literature and Medicine* 13: 1–21.

—— (1995), *The Wounded Storyteller: Body, Illness and Ethics*. Chicago: Chicago University Press.

—— (1998), Stories of illness as care of the self: A Foucauldian dialogue. *Health* 2(3): 329–348.

Franklin, Sarah (1997), *Embodied Progress: A Cultural Account of Assisted Conception*. London: Routledge.

Freund, P. and McGuire, M. (1999), Chronic illness and disability: The politics of impairment. *Health, Illness, and the Social Body: A Critical Sociology*. Upper Saddle River, NJ: Prentice-Hall, pp. 154–164.

Gafni, A., Charles, C. and Whelan, T. (1998), The physician-patient encounter: The physician as a perfect agent for the patient versus the informed treatment decision-making model. *Social Science and Medicine* 47(3): 347–354.

Gagné, P. and McGaughey, D. (2002), Designing women: Cultural hegemony and the exercise of power among women who have undergone elective mammoplasty. *Gender and Society* 16(6): 814–838.

Garrett, Catherine J. (1997), Remaking the self through metaphor: Recovery from anorexia nervosa. *Health* 1: 2, 139–156, October.

Garro, Linda (1994), Narrative representations of chronic illness experience: Cultural models of illness, mind, and body in stories concerning the temporo-mandibular joint (TMJ). *Social Science and Medicine* 38(6): 775–788.

Giddens, Anthony (1990), *The Consequences of Modernity*. Cambridge: Polity Press.

—— (1991), *Modernity and Self-Identity: Self and Society in the Late Modern Age*. Stanford, CA: Stanford University Press.

Gifford, Sandra M. (1986), The meaning of lumps: A case study of the ambiguities of risk. *Anthropology and Epidemiology: Interdisciplinary Approaches to the Study of Health and Disease*, C. Janes, R. Stall and S. Gifford (Eds). Boston: D Reidel Publishing Company, pp. 213–246.

Gill, P. S., Hunt, J. P. and Guerra, A. B. (2004), A 10-year retrospective review of 758 DIEP flaps for breast reconstruction. *Plastic and Reconstructive Surgery* 113(4): 1153–1160.

Glanz, Karen. and Lerman, Caryn (1991), Psychosocial impact of breast cancer: A critical review. *Annals of Behavioural Medicine* 14: 204–212.

Glaser, B. (1967), *The Discovery of Grounded Theory: Strategies for Qualitative Research*. New York: Aldine.

Glaser, B. and Strauss, A. (1965), *Awareness of Dying*. Chicago: Aldine.

Goffman, Erving (1956), *The Presentation of Self in Everyday Life*. Edinburgh: University of Edinburgh, Social Sciences Research Centre.

—— (1968), *Stigma: Notes on the Management of Spoiled Identity*. Harmondsworth: Penguin.

Good, Byron J. (1994), *Medicine, Rationality, and Experience: An Anthropological Perspective*. Cambridge: Cambridge University Press.

Gordon, D. and Paci, E. (1997), Disclosure practices and cultural narratives: Understanding concealment and silence around cancer in Tuscany, Italy. *Social Science and Medicine* 44(10): 1433–1452.

Gray, R., Sinding, C. and Fitch, M. (2001), Navigating the social context of metastatic breast cancer: Reflections on a project linking research to drama. *Health* 5(2): 233–248.

Grbich, Carol (1999), *Qualitative Research in Health: An Introduction*. Sydney: Allen & Unwin.

Greer, S., Morris, T. and Pettingale, K. W. (1979), Psychological response to breast cancer: Effect on outcome. *The Lancet* ii (13 October): 785–787.

Grosz, Elizabeth (1994), *Volatile Bodies: Toward a Corporeal Feminism*. St Leonards, NSW: Allen & Unwin.

Guba, E. (1996), Foreword to E. Stringer. *Action Research: A Handbook for Practitioners*. California: Sage.

Gwyn, Richard (2003), Processes of refiguration: Shifting identities in cancer narratives. *Discourse, the Body, and Identity*, J. Coupland and R. Gwyn (Eds), New York: Palgrave Macmillan (Houndmills), pp. 209–224.

Hallowell, Nina (2000), Reconstructing the body or reconstructing the woman? Problems of prophylactic mastectomy for hereditary breast cancer risk. *Ideologies of Breast Cancer: Feminist Perspectives*, L. K. Potts (Ed.). London: Macmillan Press Ltd, pp. 153–180.

Handel, N., Silverstein, M., Waisman, E. and Waisman, J. (1990), Reasons why mastectomy patients do not have breast reconstruction. *Plastic and Reconstructive Surgery* 86(6): 1118–1122.

Haraway, Donna J. (1997), *Modest_Witness@Second_Millennium.FemaleMan_ Meets_OncoMouse: Feminism and Technoscience*. New York: Routledge.

Hardey, Michael (1999), Doctor in the house: The Internet as a source of lay health knowledge and the challenge to expertise. *Sociology of Health and Illness* 21(6): 820–835.

Healy, B. (1998), Breast implants rise again – Editorial. *Journal of Women's Health* 7(6): 639–637.

Husserl, E. (1931), *Ideas I*, trans. W. Boyce Gibson. London: George Allen & Unwin.

—— (1989), *Ideas II*, trans. R. Rojcewisz and E. Schwer, W. Boyce Gibson. Dordrecht: Kluwer. First Published 1969.

Hyden, Lars-Christer (1997), Illness and narrative. *Sociology of Health and Illness* 19(1): 48–69.

Jack Watts Currie Advertising Agency (1998), National Breast Cancer Foundation advertisement for Breast Cancer Awareness Week, Australia. Personal email to S. Crompvoets, 2003.

Jacobsen, P. B. and Butler, R. W. (1996), Relation of cognitive coping and catastrophizing to acute pain and analgesic use following breast cancer surgery. *Journal of Behavioral Medicine* 19(1): 17–29, February.

Jacobson, Nora (2000), *Cleavage: Technology, Controversy, and the Ironies of the Man-Made Breast*. New Jersey: Rutgers University Press.

Jordens, C., Little, M., Paul, K. and Sayers, E.-J. (2001), Life disruption and generic complexity: A social linguistic analysis of narratives of cancer illness. *Social Science and Medicine* 53: 1227–1236.

Joss, Barbara, with Libby Harkness (1999), *My Left Breast: How Breast Cancer Transformed My Life*. Sydney: Joss & Co.

Kagawa-Singer, Marjorie (1993), Redefining health: Living with cancer. *Social Science and Medicine* 37(3): 295–304.

Kasper, Anne S. (1994), A feminist, qualitative methodology: A study of women with breast cancer. *Qualitative Sociology* 17: 263–281.

—— (1995), The social construction of breast loss and reconstruction. *Women's Health: Research on Gender, Behaviour and Policy* 1(3): 197–219.

Kaufert, Patricia A. (1998), Women, resistance, and the breast cancer movement. *Pragmatic Women and Body Politics*, M. Lock and P. Kaufert (Eds). Cambridge: Cambridge University Press. pp. 287–309.

Kavanagh, Anne, and Broom, Dorothy (1998), Embodied risk: My body, myself? *Social Science and Medicine* 46(3): 437–444.

Kellehear, A. (1993), *The Unobtrusive Researcher: A Guide to Methods*. Sydney: Allen & Unwin.

Kiefer, Carol (2001). Presenting all the choices: Teaching women about breast prosthetics (online). *Medscape Ob/Gyn & Women's Health* 6(5), http://www.medscape.com/viewarticle/408954. (Accessed 4/9/02).

Kirchgassler, K. (1990), Change and continuity in patient theories of illness: The case of epilepsy. *Social Science and Medicine* 30(12): 1313–1318.

Kissane, David, White, Kate, Cooper, Karen, and Vitetta, Louis (1999), Psychosocial support in the areas of sexuality and body image for women with breast cancer, Unpublished paper from the *Cancer We Care Conference 1999*. Sydney: NHMRC National Breast Cancer Centre.

Kitzinger, Celia (1994), The methodology of focus groups: The importance of interaction between research participants. *Sociology of Health and Illness* 16(1): 103–120.

Klawiter, Maren (2000), Racing for the cure, walking women and toxic touring: Mapping cultures of action within the Bay Area terrain of breast cancer. *Ideologies of Breast Cancer: Feminist Perspectives*, L. K. Potts (Ed.). London: Macmillan Press Ltd, pp. 63–97.

Kleinman, A., Eisenberg, L. and Good, B. (1978), Culture, illness and care: Clinical lessons from anthropologic and cross-cultural research. *Annals of Internal Medicine* 88(2): 251–258.

Kohler Riessman, Catherine (1990), Strategic uses of narrative in the presentation of self and illness: A research note. *Social Science and Medicine* 30(11): 1195–1200.

Krupat, E., Irish, J., Kasten, L., Freund, K., Burns, R., Moskowitz, M. and McKinlay, J. (1999), Patient assertiveness and physician decision-making among older breast cancer patients. *Social Science and Medicine* 49: 449–457.

Lantz, P. and Booth, K. (1998), The social construction of the breast cancer epidemic. *Social Science and Medicine* 46(7): 907–918.

Leopold, Ellen (1999), *A Darker Ribbon: Breast Cancer, Women, and Their Doctors in the Twentieth Century*. Boston: Beacon Press.

Lerner, Baron (2000), Inventing a curable disease: Historical perspectives on breast cancer. *Breast Cancer: Society Shapes an Epidemic*, A. Kasper and S. Ferguson (Eds). New York: St Martin's Press, pp. 25–50.

Little Miles (2004), Chronic illness and the experience of surviving cancer. *Internal Medicine Journal* 34(4): 201–202, April.

Little, M., Jordens, C., Paul, K., Montgomery, K. and Philipson, B. (1998), Liminality: A major category of the experience of cancer illness. *Social Science and Medicine* 47(10): 1485–1494.

Little, M., Paul, K., Jordens, C. and Sayers, E.-J. (2000), Vulnerability in the narratives of patients and their carers: Studies of colo-rectal cancer. *Health* 4(4): 499–514.

Lock, Margaret (1998), Breast cancer: Reading the omens. *Anthropology Today* 14(4): 7–16.

Lorde, Audre (1980), The Cancer Journals, reprinted in *The Audre Lorde Compendium: Essays, Speeches and Journals* (1996), London: Pandora, pp. 1–64.

Lowrey, Phillipa (1990), Breast augmentation. *Proceedings of the Women and Surgery Conference 1990*, R. Moore (Ed.). Melbourne: HealthSharing Women, pp. 74–82.

Lupton, Deborah (1994a), *Medicine as Culture: Illness, Disease and the Body in Western Societies*. London: Sage.

—— (1994b), Femininity, responsibility, and the technological imperative: Discourses on breast cancer in the Australian press. *International Journal of Health Services* 24(1): 73–89.

Malson, Helen (1998), *The Thin Woman: Feminism, Post-Structuralism and the Social Psychology of Anorexia Nervosa*. London: Routledge.

Manderson, Lenore (1999), Gender, normality and the post-surgical body. *Anthropology and Medicine* 6(3): 381–394.

Martin, Emily (1987), *The Woman in the Body*. Boston, Massachusetts: Beacon Press.

Mathieson, Cynthia. and Stam, Henderikus (1995), Renegotiating identity: Cancer narratives. *Sociology of Health and Illness* 17(3): 283–306.

Matuschka (1993), Beauty out of damage, in Cartwright, Lisa (1998), Community and the public body in breast cancer media activism. *Cultural Studies* 12(2): 125.

McKay, S. and Bonner, F. (1999), Telling stories: Breast cancer pathographies in Australian women's magazines. *Women's Studies International Forum* 22(5): 563–571.

McQueen, D. (1999), A world behaving badly: The global challenge for behavioural surveillance. *American Journal of Public Health* 89(9): 1312–1314.

Mechanic, D. (1968), *Medical Sociology*. New York: Free Press.

Meyerowitz, B. E. (1980), Psychosocial correlates of breast cancer and its treatments. *Psychological Bulletin* 87: 108–131.

Miller, G. and Dingwell, R. (1997), *Context and Method in Qualitative Research*. London: Sage Publications.

Minichiello, V., Aroni, R., Timewell., E. and Alexander, L. (1995), *In-Depth Interviewing, Second Edition*. Australia: Longman.

Mock, V. (1993), Body image in women treated for breast cancer. *Nursing Research* 42(30): 153–157.

Mol, Annemarie (1998), Missing links, making links: The performance of some Atheroscleroses. *Differences in Medicine: Unravelling Practices, Techniques, and Bodies*, M. Berg and A. Mol (Eds). London: Duke University Press.

—— (1999), Ontological politics. A word and some questions. *Actor Network Theory and After*, J. Law and J. Hassard (Eds). Oxford: Blackwell Publishers, pp. 74–89.

Montini, T. (1996), Gender and emotion in the advocacy of breast cancer informed consent legislation. *Gender and Society* 10: 9–23.

Murcott, A. (1981), On the typification of bad patients. *Medical Work, Realities and Routines*, P. Atkinson and C. Heath (Eds). London: Gower, pp. 128–140.

National Breast Cancer Foundation (2002), *Pink Ribbon*. Sydney, Australia: National Breast Cancer Foundation.

National Health & Medical Research Council (1995), *A Consumer's Guide: Early Breast Cancer*. NSW: NHMRC.

—— (1996), *All About Early Breast Cancer*. Australia: NHMRC.

NSW Breast Cancer Institute (1999a), Risk factors for breast cancer (online), *NSW Breast Cancer Institute*, http://www.bci.org.au/public/facts2.htm (Accessed 9/9/03).

—— (1999b), Trends in incidence and mortality (online), *NSW Breast Cancer Institute*, http://www.bci.org.au/public/facts3.htm (Accessed 9/9/03).

Oakley, Ann (1981), Interviewing women – a contradiction in terms. *Doing Feminist Research*, H. Roberts (Ed.). London: Routledge & Kegan Paul.

Opie, Anne (1992), *There's Nobody There: Community Care of Confused Older People*. Auckland: Oxford University Press.

Orbach, S. (1988), *Fat is a Feminist Issue*. London: Arrow Books.

Parker, Lisa S. (1995), Beauty and breast implantation: How candidate selection affects autonomy and informed consent. *Hypatia* 10(1): 183–201.

Parsons, Talcott (1951), *The Social System*. London: Routledge & Kegan Paul.

Pascoe, S. W., Neal, R. D., Allgar, V. L., Selby P. J. and Wright, E. P. (2004), Psychosocial care for cancer patients in primary care? Recognition of opportunities for cancer care. *Family Practice* 21(4):437–442.

Paszat, L. F., Groome, P. A. and Schulze, K. (2000), A population-based study of the effectiveness of breast conservation for newly diagnosed breast cancer. *International Journal of Radiation Oncology Biology Physics* 46(2): 345–353.

Pauly Morgan, Kathryn (1991), Women and the knife: Cosmetic surgery and the colonisation of women's bodies. *Hypatia* 6(3): 25–53.

Pennington, David (1999), Reconstructions: Expert opinions. *My Left Breast: How Breast Cancer Transformed My Life*, B. Joss (Ed.). Sydney: Joss & Co., pp. 127–134.

Peto, R. (1998), Mortality from breast cancer in UK has decreased suddenly. *British Medical Journal* 317: 476–477.

—— (2000), UK and USA breast cancer deaths down 25% in year 2000 at ages 20–69 years. *Lancet* 355: 1822.

Pettingale, K. W., Morris, T., Greer, S. and Haybittle, J. L. (1985), Mental attitudes to cancer: An additional prognostic factor. *Lancet* (March 30): 750.

Pierce, P. F. (1993), Deciding on breast cancer treatment: A description of decision-making behaviour. *Nursing Research* 42(22): 22–28.

Price, B. (1992), Living with altered body image: The cancer experience. *British Journal of Nursing* 1(3): 641–645.

Queensland Cancer Fund (2000), *A Guide for the Partners of Women with Breast Cancer: How to Help*. Qld, Australia: Queensland Cancer Fund.

Radley, Alan and Billig, Michael (1996), Accounts of health and illness: Dilemmas and representations. *Sociology of Health and Illness* 18(2): 220–240.

Reaby, Linda L., Hort, Linda K. and Vandervord, John (1994), Body image, self-concept, and self-esteem in women who had a mastectomy and either wore an external breast prosthesis or had breast reconstruction and women who had not experienced mastectomy. *Health Care for Women International* 15: 361–375.

Reaby, Linda L. (1996), *Post-Mastectomy Self-Perceptions, Attitudes and Breast Restoration Decision-Making*. Canberra: University of Canberra.
—— (1998a), Breast restoration decision making: Enhancing the process. *Cancer Nursing* 21(3): 196–204.
—— (1998b), Reasons why women who have mastectomy decide to have or not to have breast reconstruction. *Plastic and Reconstructive Surgery* 101(7): 1810–1818.
—— (1999), Breast restoration decision making. *Plastic Surgical Nursing* 19(1): 22–30.
Reaby, Linda L. and Hort, Linda K. (1995), Post-mastectomy attitudes in women who wear external breast prostheses compared to those who have undergone breast reconstructions. *Journal of Behavioural Medicine* 18(1): 55–67.
Redman, S., Turner, J. and Davis, C. (2003), Improving supportive care for women with breast cancer in Australia: The challenge of modifying health systems. *Psycho-Oncology* 12(6): 521–531, September.
Rees, G., Fry, A. and Cull, A. (2001), A family history of breast cancer: Women's experiences from a theoretical perspective. *Social Science and Medicine* 52: 1433–1440.
Reynolds, J. S. and Perrin, N. A. (2004), Mismatches in social support and psychosocial adjustment to breast cancer. *Health Psychology* 23(4): 425–430, July.
Roberts, Celia (2000), Training women to be critical: Breast cancer consumer advocacy and science training workshops. Unpublished paper from the *Anti-Cancer Council Feminist Approaches to Breast Cancer Conference 2000*, Carlton, Melbourne.
Robertson, Ann (2001), Biotechnology, political rationality and discourses on health risk. *Health* 5(3): 293–310.
Robinson, Ian (1990), Personal narratives, social careers and medical courses: Analysing life trajectories in autobiographies of people with multiple sclerosis. *Social Science and Medicine* 30(11): 1173–1186.
Rosenbaum, Marcy and Roos, Gun (2000), Women's experiences of breast cancer. *Breast Cancer: Society Shapes an Epidemic*, A. Kasper and S. Ferguson (Eds). New York: St Martin's Press, pp. 153–182.
Rowland, J., Dioso, J., Holland, J., Chaglassian, T. and Kinne, D. (1995), Breast reconstruction after mastectomy: Who seeks it, who refuses? *Plastic and Reconstructive Surgery* 95(5): 812–822.
Royal Women's Hospital (2002), Women's art @whic (online), *Wellwomen's website*, http://www.rwh.org.au/wellwomens/whic.cfm?doc_id=2446 (Accessed 10/9/03).
Saillant, Francine (1990), Discourse, knowledge and experience of cancer: A life story. *Culture, Medicine and Psychiatry* 14: 81–104.
Saywell, C., Henderson, L. and Beattie, L. (2000), Sexualised illness: The newsworthy body in media representations of breast cancer. *Ideologies of Breast Cancer: Feminist Perspectives*, L. K. Potts (Ed.). London: Macmillan Press Ltd, pp. 37–62.
Scanlon, Edward F. (1991), The role of reconstruction in breast cancer. *Cancer* 68(5): 1144–1147.
Sered, Susan and Tabory, Ephraim (1999), 'You are a number, not a human being': Israeli breast cancer patients' experiences with the medical establishment. *Medical Anthropology Quarterly* 13(2): 223–252.
Shaffir, W. B., Stebbins, R. A. and Turowetz, A. (1980), *Fieldwork Experience: Qualitative Approaches to Social Research*. London: Routledge & Kegan Paul.
Shain, W., Wellisch, D., Pasnau, R. and Landsverk, J. (1985), The sooner the better: A study of psychological factors in undergoing immediate versus delayed breast reconstruction. *American Journal of Psychiatry* 142(40): 40–46.

Sharf, Barbara F. (1997), Communicating breast cancer on-line: Support and empowerment on the internet. *Women & Health* 26(1): 65–84.

Silverman, David (1987), *Communication and Medical Practice: Social Relations in the Clinic*. London: Sage.

Simpson, Christy (2000), Controversies in breast cancer prevention: The discourse of risk. *Ideologies of Breast Cancer: Feminist Perspectives*, L. K. Potts (Ed.). London: Macmillan Press Ltd, pp. 131–152.

Singletary, S. E. (2001) New approaches to surgery for breast cancer. *Endocrine-Related Cancer* 8(4): 265–286, December.

Smith, D. E. (1990), *Texts, Facts and Femininity: Exploring the Relations of Ruling*. London: Routledge.

Sontag, Susan (1978). *Illness as Metaphor*. New York: Farrar, Straus & Giroux.

—— (1989), *AIDS and Its Metaphors*. New York: Farrar, Straus & Giroux.

Stacey, Jackie (1997), *Teratologies: A Cultural Study of Cancer*. London: Routledge.

Stanley, Liz and Wise, Sue (1983), *Breaking Out: Feminist Consciousness and Feminist Research*. London: Routledge & Kegan Paul.

Stevens, Joyce (1995), *Healing Women: A History of Leichhardt Women's Community Health Centre*. Leichhardt, NSW: First Ten Years History Project.

Strauss, A. (1987), *Qualitative Analysis for Social Scientists*. London: Cambridge University Press.

Taylor, C. (1996), *Sources of the Self: The Making of Modern Identity*. Cambridge: Cambridge University Press.

Taylor, S. E. (1983), Adjustment to threatening events: A theory of cognitive adaptation. *American Psychologist* 58: 1161–1173.

—— (1989), *Positive Illusions: Creative Self-Deception and the Healthy Mind*. New York: Basic Books.

—— (1990), Health psychology: The science and the field. *American Psychologist* 45: 40–50.

Taylor, V. and Van Willigen, M. (1996), Women's self help and the reconstruction of gender: The postpartum support and breast cancer movements. *Mobilization: An International Journal* 1: 123–143.

The Australian Society of Plastic Surgeons (2001), Breast reconstruction after mastectomy (online), *ASPS website*, http://www.plasticsurgery.org.au/public/aspsframe.asp. (Accessed 5/7/03).

Thewes, B., Butow, P. and Girgis, A. (2004) The psychosocial needs of breast cancer survivors: A qualitative study of the shared and unique needs of younger versus older survivors. *Psycho-Oncology* 13(3): 177–189, March.

Thorne, S. and Murray, C. (2000), Social constructions of breast cancer. *Health Care for Women International* 21: 141–159.

Tulloh, B. and Goldsworthy, M. (1997), Breast cancer management: A rural perspective (online). *Medical Journal of Australia Online*, http://www.mja.com.au (Accessed 10/9/99).

Turner, Bryan S. (1992), *Regulating Bodies: Essays in Medical Sociology*. USA: Routledge.

—— (1995), *Medical Power and Social Knowledge, Second edition*. London: Sage.

Ussher, Jane (1992), Reproductive rhetoric and the blaming of the body. *The Psychology of Women's Health and Health Care*, P. Nicholson and J. Ussher (Eds). London: Macmillan Press Ltd, pp. 31–61.

van der Molen, B. (2000), Relating information needs to the cancer experience: Jenny's story – a cancer narrative. *European Journal of Cancer Care* 7(1): 41–47.

Wainstock, J. M. (1991), Breast cancer: Psychosocial consequences for the patient. *Seminars in Oncology Nursing* 7: 207–215.

Wardlow, H. and Curry, R. (1996), 'Sympathy for my body': Breast cancer and mammography at two Atlanta clinics. *Medical Anthropology* 16: 319–340.

Waxler-Morrison, N., Doll, R. and Hislop, G. (1995), The use of qualitative methods to strengthen psychosocial research on cancer. *Journal of Psychosocial Oncology* 13: 177–191.

White, Kevin (2002), *The Sociology of Health and Illness*. London and New York: Sage.

Wickman, M. (1995), Breast reconstruction – Past achievements, current status and future goals. *Scandinavian Journal of Plastic and Reconstructive Hand Surgery* 29: 81–100.

Wijsbek, H. (2000), The pursuit of beauty: The enforcement of aesthetics or a freely adopted lifestyle? *Journal of Medical Ethics* 26(6): 454–458.

Wilkinson, Sue (1998), Focus groups in feminist research: Power, interaction, and the co-construction of meaning. *Women's Studies International Forum* 21(1): 111–125.

—— (2000), Feminist research traditions in health psychology: Breast cancer research. *Journal of Health Psychology* 5(3): 359–372.

—— (2001), Breast cancer: Feminism, representations and resistance: A commentary on Dorothy Broom's 'Reading Breast Cancer'. *Health* 5(2): 269–278.

Wilkinson, Sue and Kitzinger, Celia (1994), Towards a feminist approach to breast cancer. *Women and Health: Feminist Perspectives*, S. Wilkinson and C. Kitzinger (Eds). London: Taylor & Francis.

—— (2000), Thinking differently about thinking positive: A discursive approach to breast cancer patients talk. *Social Science and Medicine* 50: 797–811.

Williams, Gareth (1984), The genesis of chronic illness: Narrative re-construction. *Sociology of Health and Illness* 6(2): 175–200.

Williams, Simon J. (1997), Modern medicine and the 'uncertain body': From corporeality to hyperreality? *Social Science and Medicine* 45(7): 1041–1949.

Woman's Day (1998), 'You have to shock people': Barbara's brave battle. *Woman's Day* 2 November, 1998. Sydney, NSW: ACP Publishing Pty Ltd.

Yadlon, Susan (1997), Skinny women and good mothers: The rhetoric of risk, control and culpability in the production of knowledge about breast cancer. *Feminist Studies* 23(3): 645–677.

Young, Iris Marion (1990), *Throwing Like a Girl and Other Essays in Feminist Philosophy and Social Theory*. Bloomington: Indiana University Press.

Index